Hospital Management and Administration - Improving the Quality of Health Services

Edited by Hatice Esen Koç and Nazife Öztürk

Published in London, United Kingdom

Hospital Management and Administration - Improving the Quality of Health Services
http://dx.doi.org/10.5772/intechopen.1006012
Edited by Hatice Esen Koç and Nazife Öztürk

Contributors
Hatice Esen Koc, Hatice Esen Koç, Matthew Mazurek, Nazife Ozturk, Pir Hossein Kolivand, Ömer Faruk Sağlam

First published in London, United Kingdom, 2026 by IntechOpen
IntechOpen is the global imprint of INTECHOPEN LIMITED, registered in England and Wales, registration number: 11086078, 167-169 Great Portland Street, London, W1W 5PF, United Kingdom

For EU product safety concerns: IN TECH d.o.o., Prolaz Marije Krucifikse Kozulić 3, 51000 Rijeka, Croatia, info@intechopen.com or visit our website at intechopen.com.

British Library Cataloguing-in-Publication Data
A catalogue record for this book is available from the British Library

Hospital Management and Administration - Improving the Quality of Health Services
Edited by Hatice Esen Koç and Nazife Öztürk
p. cm.

This title is part of the Public Health Book Series, Volume 13
Topic: Healthcare and Management
Series Editor: José Antonio Mirón Canelo
Topic Editor: Aida Isabel Tavares

Print ISBN 978-1-83635-025-5
Online ISBN 978-1-83635-024-8
eBook (PDF) ISBN 978-1-83635-026-2
ISSN 3049-8872

IntechOpen Book Series
Public Health
Volume 13

Aims and Scope of the Series

Public health is what we as a society do collectively to contribute to and ensure the health and social conditions for the enjoyment of health as a resource for life. It can also be defined as science and research that promotes health, prevents disease, and improves populations' well-being and quality of life. Its objective is to know the risk factors that determine and condition the populations' health levels at present. At the end of the 20th century and the beginning of the 21st century, it is unjustifiable and regrettable that morbimortality according to age plays a leading role when the causes are mostly well known and therefore preventable, such as obesity, AIDS, cirrhosis, diabetes mellitus, addictions and cancer associated with the consumption of tobacco and alcohol, etc. In short, public health is science based on epidemiology and biostatistics, and currently, new technologies and artificial intelligence must be incorporated to identify patterns and trends in what we do collectively as a society to ensure living conditions and prevent risk factors that affect individual and population health. For all these reasons, it is essential to scientifically investigate and act on the determinants that impede the well-being and quality of life related to the health of people, patients, and populations in general, given that to control the determinants of diseases, it is important to control the environment and genetics. Consequently, the current fight for public health must prioritize the control of the environment, such as atmospheric and biological pollution and environmental and social biodiversity, promoting the sensitivity and training of society and its individuals by empowering them to make free and appropriate decisions about these aspects to lead healthy lifestyles based on motivation and responsibility in the face of the challenges they cope with from an individual point of view, such as dealing with the addictions that exist in today's complex world. Public health also requires an ethical vision and incorporates strategies to reduce social inequality.

Meet the Series Editor

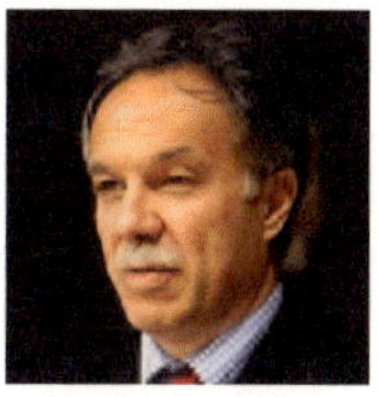

José Antonio Mirón Canelo is a physician, doctor, and professor of Preventive Medicine and Public Health at the Faculty of Medicine and Dentistry of the University of Salamanca with over 30 years of experience. He is the director of the USAL's Expert Degree in Health Management, currently in its 13th edition. Prof. Mirón Canelo directs a research group at the Research Institute of Biomedical Sciences (IBSAL) of the University of Salamanca focused on addressing the challenges and care needs of vulnerable people and patients such as the elderly with multiple pathologies and people with disabilities and dependence. As a teacher, he has been recognized for excellence in teaching three times in a period of five years.

Meet the Volume Editors

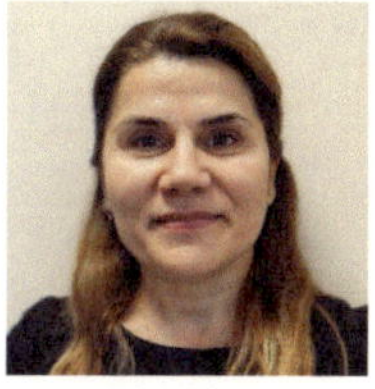

Hatice Esen Koç graduated from Akdeniz University in 1999, completed her master's degree in Internal Medicine Nursing at Afyon Kocatepe University in 2008, and received her Ph.D. in Health Management from Süleyman Demirel University in 2019. She became an Associate Professor in 2024. Her research primarily focuses on quality and accreditation in healthcare, as well as on efficiency and performance management in healthcare institutions. She has presented papers, published articles, and presented at national and international symposiums in her areas of expertise. Additionally, she has participated in numerous national and international projects, contributing to the development of knowledge in her field. She has published extensively in health management, with more than 30 peer-reviewed publications to her credit, including two book chapters and one edited book. She currently works in the R&D unit of Antalya Training and Research Hospital.

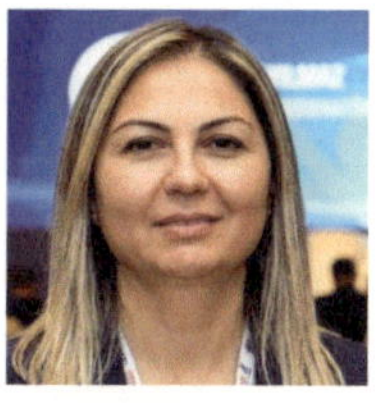

Assoc. Prof. Dr. Nazife Öztürk holds a bachelor's and master's degree in Health Management from Ankara University. She earned her Ph.D. in Health Administration from Süleyman Demirel University in 2019. Currently, she serves as an Associate Professor within the Research and Development Department at Antalya Training and Research Hospital. Her academic portfolio focuses on health management and its interdisciplinary applications. Dr. Öztürk has contributed extensively to the field, with over 25 peer-reviewed publications and two book chapters to her credit. Beyond her publications, she has actively engaged in numerous national and international projects and frequently presents her research at global congresses through both oral and poster presentations.

Contents

Preface

Healthcare delivery has been based on a continuous patient-physician relationship since its inception, and today it encompasses the relationship and collaboration of multidisciplinary healthcare professionals. The principle of "first, do no harm" (Primum non nocere) remains the fundamental cornerstone in healthcare delivery, guiding every clinical and administrative decision. Therefore, the importance of healthcare services for individuals' physical, emotional, and mental well-being, based on recorded health information and the expert assistance of healthcare professionals, is immense. In the modern era, quality in healthcare delivery and the efficient use of patient life expectancy are vital. Patients must not only receive treatment but also feel safe within the healthcare ecosystem. However, informing patients is no longer enough to win their trust; patient safety values must be continuously maintained and integrated into all components of healthcare services, from front-line clinical care to back-office administration. With rapid technological advancements and digital transformations, hospital management has undergone a paradigm shift from traditional hierarchical management to alternative, visionary, and data-driven management. Therefore, hospital support systems and administrative frameworks must adapt to the innovations of the era, ensuring the efficient use of existing resources while maintaining high standards of care. This book, "Hospital Management and Administration – Improving the Quality of Health Services", brings together comprehensive theoretical knowledge and diverse practical applications in hospital management and patient safety. As editors, we aimed to provide the reader with both a robust general framework and the necessary depth of detail by bringing together important topics from an interdisciplinary perspective. Each chapter explores different facets of the evolving landscape, offering insights into how visionary leadership can address contemporary challenges in the healthcare sector. We would like to thank all the chapter authors for their expertise. We believe this work contributes significantly to hospital management and patient safety, benefiting all stakeholders in health services.

Dr. Hatice Esen Koç and Dr. Nazife Öztürk
Associate Professor,
Antalya Training and Research Hospital,
R&D Unit,
Antalya, Türkiye

Chapter 1

Introductory Chapter: An Overview of Healthcare Service Quality

Hatice Esen Koç

1. Introduction

The continuous provision of healthcare services 7/24 is indispensable and of vital importance for the well-being of individuals and societies. Hospital management plays a pivotal role in delivering high-quality healthcare services, ensuring the efficient use of all available resources, and maintaining accessibility. In today's world, rising healthcare expenditures, an ageing population, the increasing prevalence of chronic diseases, technological advancements, and rising patient expectations have rendered hospital management—with its matrix organisational structure—more complex and strategically demanding [1, 2].

The World Health Organisation (WHO) defines quality healthcare services as those that are *effective*, *safe*, *people-centred*, *timely*, *equitable*, *integrated*, and *efficient* [3]. For healthcare services to be considered high quality, they must achieve the objectives outlined above. Within the scope of healthcare services, the *health quality standards (HQS)* have been established in alignment with the WHO patient safety objectives to ensure quality assurance in hospitals. These standards include the following targets: effectiveness, efficiency, productivity, healthy working life, patient safety, equity, patient-centredness, convenience, timeless, and continuity [4]. The *Türkiye* Quality and Accreditation in Health (*TUSKA*) plays a crucial role in ensuring that hospitals comply with national and international standards and in establishing a culture of continuous improvement [5].

The healthcare accreditation standards demonstrate alignment with the patient safety goals set out by the World Health Organisation (**Figure 1**).

A patient-centred approach is critical for ensuring patient safety and satisfaction. Since the 1980s, there has been recognition of the potential of a patient-centred healthcare system to offer significant opportunities for hospitals to improve their quality and, consequently, their efficiency [6]. Today, hospital managers are required not only to ensure operational efficiency but also to demonstrate competence in strategic leadership, financial sustainability, digital transformation, human resources management, and risk management. In this context, traditional hospital management has evolved beyond classical administrative duties into a multidisciplinary leadership role.

1.1 Hospital management of the future

The accessibility and sustainability of healthcare services is of critical importance. In the healthcare sector, effective leadership is crucial for the effective management of resources and the success of healthcare operations. In healthcare institutions, it is not only about managing existing resources; effective green leadership that focuses

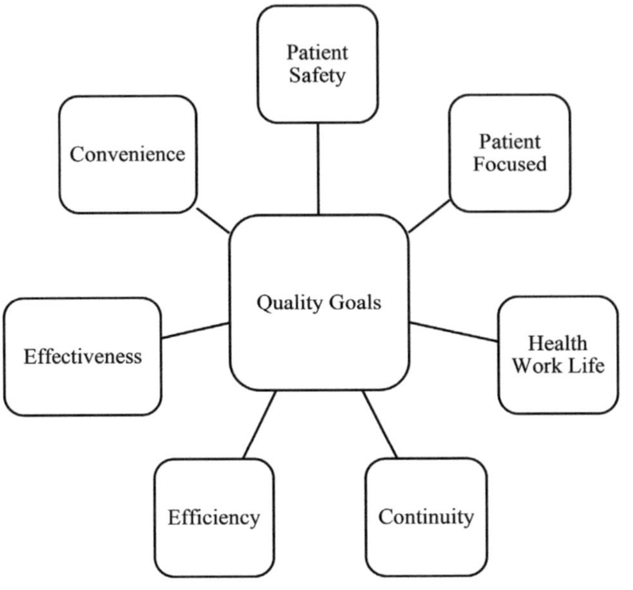

Figure 1.
HQS goals (TUSKA).

on social and environmental responsibility, as well as visionary leadership grounded in ethical values and mindful of the balance of the environmental ecosystem, is of paramount importance [7]. The issue of sustainability assumes particular significance in the context of hospitals, primarily in order to fulfil social requirements and to avoid environmental and health risks. Moreover, in consequence of the considerable technological and digital changes and transformations that have occurred in the recent years, it is imperative for healthcare institutions to adopt innovation and to implement approach that are innovative, if strategic development is to be achieved [8].

The necessity for high-quality, accessible, and affordable healthcare services is increasing in line with population growth, an ageing society, and the increasing prevalence of chronic diseases. These challenges are compelling healthcare systems to develop more efficient, sustainable, and innovative solutions. This necessitates creative approaches to health economics, social policy, and effective management to ensure the delivery of high-quality services. The existence of successful and sustainable healthcare systems is predicated on technological advancements and the utilisation of evidence-based research.

Another important aspect of healthcare is Industry 4.0, the digital revolution of the twenty-first century. This has led to the creation of a "Healthcare 4.0" system, a summary of future technologies that aims to make healthcare systems more efficient, personalised, and sustainable. Protecting against an ageing population and increasing chronic diseases, technologies such as real-time data collection, AI-powered predictive analytics, and telemedicine provide early diagnosis, personalised treatment, and resource planning. The COVID-19 pandemic highlighted the urgency of this digitalization, emphasising the increasing need for stronger and more adaptable healthcare outcomes [9].

The primary responsibility of current hospital administrators is to ensure patient safety when providing quality healthcare, while also prioritising environmental and social sustainability, integrating digital transformation, and constructing more efficient, personalised healthcare systems for the future.

DOI: http://dx.doi.org/10.5772/intechopen.1015798

2. Purpose and goals

In editing this book, a clear mission was set: to provide a state-of-the-art look at the hospital management and patient safety. The challenges and complexities of hospital management are highlighted by this text; the integrity of traditional hospital management roles is emphasised; the concept of visionary leadership is outlined; the digital transformation of healthcare is outlined; the quality of healthcare is outlined, as well as patient safety, accessibility, and sustainability; and the delivery of more effective and efficient healthcare services is emphasised, with a patient-centred approach throughout this process. In this regard, adopting a holistic approach to the delivery of quality healthcare services centred on patient safety is of paramount importance.

3. Conclusion

At its core, this book offers solutions to current health problems, it also discusses future product options. Furthermore, it emphasises the importance of ethical values and patient-centred methods in healthcare management, guiding service delivery within the sector. It is vital that practices aimed at ensuring patient safety and continuously improving healthcare delivery be supported by effective hospital management. In particular, the hospital support provided today should adopt and implement a comprehensive visionary perspective, encompassing patient and staff safety, patient and staff satisfaction, risk management, learning from mistakes, and continuous quality control. I would like to express my sincere gratitude to all my colleagues and contributors who worked on the preparation of this book.

Acknowledgements

The author acknowledges the use of Grok AI for the language polishing of the chapter.

Author details

Hatice Esen Koç
Antalya Training and Research Hospital, Antalya, Türkiye

*Address all correspondence to: hatice.esen@gmail.com

References

[1] Ward C et al. What is the relationship between hospital management practices and quality of care? A systematic review of the global evidence. Health Policy and Planning. 2025;**40**(3):409-421. DOI: 10.1093/heapol/czae112

[2] Endalamaw A et al. A scoping review of continuous quality improvement in healthcare system: Conceptualization, models and tools, barriers and facilitators, and impact. BMC Health Services Research. 2024;**24**:487. DOI: 10.1186/s12913-024-10828-0

[3] World Health Organization. Quality Health Services. Geneva: WHO; 2023. Available from: https://www.who.int/news-room/fact-sheets/detail/quality-health-services

[4] Health Quality Standards (HQS). Hospital (Version 6.1). Ankara: Türkiye Ministry of Health, General Directorate of Health Services, Department of Quality, Accreditation and Employee Rights in Healthcare; 2020. Available from: https://shgm.saglik.gov.tr

[5] Türkiye Health Care Quality and Accreditation Institute (TUSKA). Quality and Accreditation in Health Hospital Set. Ankara: Türkiye Ministry of Health; 2024. Available from: https://tuska.tuseb.gov.tr

[6] Perals PO, Rambaud SC, Garcíal JS. Quality of care and patient satisfaction: Future trends and economic implications for the healthcare system 2025. Journal of Economic Surveys. 2025;**39**:1327-1360. DOI: 10.1111/joes.12657

[7] Bevere D, Faccilongo N. Shaping the future of healthcare: Integrating ecology and digital innovation. Sustainability. 2024;**2024**(16):3835. DOI: 10.3390/su16093835

[8] Lopes CM et al. Perspective of business models and innovation for sustainability transition in hospitals. Sustainability. 2019;**11**:5. DOI: 10.3390/su11010005

[9] Ferreira ARO, Tiago A, Fernandes TA. Innovating for tomorrow: Industry 4.0's role in sustainable healthcare. Health and Technology. 2026;**16**:59-71. DOI: 10.1007/s12553-025-01050-x

Chapter 2

Perspective Chapter: The Strategic Importance of Professionalism in Healthcare

Hatice Esen Koc and Nazife Öztürk

Abstract

Professionalism is widely recognized as a fundamental component of high-quality, safe, and patient-centered healthcare. It encompasses a set of values, behaviors, and relationships that support the public's trust in healthcare professionals. In the context of contemporary hospital management, the promotion of professionalism is not only an ethical imperative but also a strategic necessity. Health systems are becoming increasingly complex, multidisciplinary, and results-oriented. In such environments, professionalism serves both as a guiding principle and a performance enhancer. This section explores the concept of professionalism as a multifaceted and evolving phenomenon that extends beyond individual healthcare providers to encompass organizational structures, leadership methodologies, and organizational culture. The concept of professionalism is presented as a strategic tool that contributes to organizational excellence, staff loyalty, ethical decision-making, and ultimately improved patient outcomes. The present section has been prepared using academic literature and international frameworks. The objective of this study is to furnish healthcare managers, policymakers, and educators with pragmatic insights into the development, sustenance, and integration of professionalism into the fundamental operations of healthcare delivery.

Keywords: healthcare, professionalism, healthcare quality, healthcare management, hospital management

1. Introduction

Healthcare institutions are under significant pressure to improve their services due to an aging population and increasing demand for healthcare services. The development of the human qualities of healthcare professionals is of crucial importance in ensuring the provision of high-quality medical service [1]. The cornerstone of patient-centered, reliable, and ethical service delivery in healthcare is professionalism. Within the context of clinical settings, professional conduct is regarded not only as an individual responsibility but also as a metric by which to gauge organizational performance. In the contemporary context of hospital management, a strategic approach to professionalism is imperative, given the complex structure of modern hospitals, the multidisciplinary nature of their teams, and their emphasis on patient satisfaction [2]. The provision of safe, effective, patient-centered, timely, efficient, and equitable clinical care is dependent on medical professionalism. The fundamental principles of medical professionalism are firmly entrenched within the historical context, as evidenced by the existence of oaths and established expectations [3]. Consequently, the concept of professionalism transcends individual values and ethics, being instead closely associated with institutional leadership, policies, employee development strategies, and organizational culture. In this context, the adoption of a professional approach has been demonstrated to enhance the quality of healthcare services while concomitantly strengthening employee job satisfaction and commitment [4]. Consequently, promoting professionalism is imperative for the sustainable success of healthcare institutions. The notion of professionalism in healthcare services is predicated on the existence of an effective human resources policy, which must be continuously developed. This approach has the potential to enhance patient satisfaction and strengthen the motivation of healthcare workers. Furthermore, cultivating professionalism is a pivotal strategy for navigating the intricacies of the healthcare system and enhancing the efficacy of multidisciplinary teams.

1.1 Definition and development of professionalism

The concept of professionalism has historically been defined within the framework of the medical profession's contract with society. This contract is predicated on a set of principles, including knowledge, ethical values, dedication, and prioritization of the public interest [5]. In contemporary discourse, the concept of professionalism is understood in conjunction with the notion of organizational professionalism, superseding individual attitudes. Clinical professionalism is defined as the behaviors of physicians and nurses who are in direct contact with patients. In contrast, managerial professionalism refers to institutional practices such as leadership approach, strategic decision-making, transparency, and accountability. In this context, the development of professionalism is a crucial strategic goal for enhancing the quality of healthcare delivery and motivating healthcare workers. The notion of professionalism in healthcare is predicated on the existence of an effective human resources policy that is subject to continuous development. This will increase patient satisfaction and strengthen the motivation of healthcare workers. In this context, the constant strengthening of professionalism is a critical strategy for adapting to the complexity of the healthcare system and increasing the effectiveness of multidisciplinary teams. The concept of professionalism is inherently dynamic, necessitating continuous development at both the individual and institutional levels within healthcare services. The impact of professionalism on healthcare services has the potential to improve patient outcomes and optimize healthcare delivery. In this context, the development of professionalism emerges as a critical strategy for adapting to the complexity of the healthcare system and increasing the effectiveness of multidisciplinary teams. In conclusion, professionalism can be defined as a dynamic process that can improve the quality of healthcare services. Furthermore, it has been demonstrated that it can also strengthen employee job satisfaction and commitment.

Academic environments that facilitate the imparting of medical education and professional values have been shown to play a critical role in the development of professionalism. Papadakis and colleagues [6] demonstrated that deviations from professionalism in medical school education increase the likelihood of disciplinary action later in one's professional life. This underscores the imperative for the initiation of professional education at an early stage, with due emphasis placed on its uninterrupted progression. In academic education processes, ethical sensitivity, empathy development, and the encouragement of professional attitudes through motivational elements facilitate the transformation of professionalism into a lifelong behavioral pattern [6].

Furthermore, the necessity for a clear definition of corporate values and their alignment with the workplace culture arises from the differences in employees' perceptions of professionalism [7]. The establishment of an organizational culture characterized by professionalism is predicated on the presence of internal policies, the formulation of behavioral standards, and the implementation of mechanisms for the monitoring of compliance with these standards. To achieve this objective, all employees must embrace corporate values within the framework of transparency, fairness, and professional contract principles.

The concept of institutional professionalism extends beyond mere behavioral aspects, encompassing leadership methodologies, ethical decision-making processes, and reward systems. Edgar [5] posits that the design of institutional structures that foster professional conduct among employees has the potential to enhance their motivation levels and the quality of the services they deliver. It is evident that a professional approach, endorsed by corporate policies, exerts a favorable influence on employee loyalty, patient satisfaction, and organizational performance.

To adapt to the constantly changing dynamics of healthcare systems, professional principles must be supported by flexibility and innovation. The contemporary healthcare environment is characterized by several factors that are forcing a redefinition of the concept of professionalism. These factors include multidisciplinary work environments, increasing patient diversity, and digital transformation. The result of these developments is that professionalism is becoming increasingly inclusive [8]. The concept of professionalism must be subject to continuous updating and development, both on an individual level, through the personal professional values of individuals, and on an institutional level, through the implementation of institutional strategies.

The fundamental structural elements of professionalism in healthcare services are demonstrated in **Figure 1**. It is crucial to emphasize that these essential elements are indispensable for achieving true professionalism in healthcare services.

1.2 Dimensions of professionalism in healthcare institutions

The concept of professionalism is manifested in diverse dimensions at the individual, team, and institutional levels. At the individual level, the following measures are recommended: Internalizing one's professional identity, demonstrating commitment to ethical values, and respecting patient rights are of paramount importance.

At the team level, the following elements are particularly significant in this context: multidisciplinary work, cooperation, mutual respect, and effective communication.

At the institutional level, the following observations can be made: it is imperative to implement policies that encourage professional behavior, leadership approach, performance evaluation, and education systems.

These dimensions interact with each other, and they must be addressed collectively to ensure the continuity of institutional professionalism. In this context, healthcare institutions must formulate strategic plans to enhance their understanding of professionalism and provide continuous education programs to advance the skills of their employees. The implementation of these strategic plans has the potential

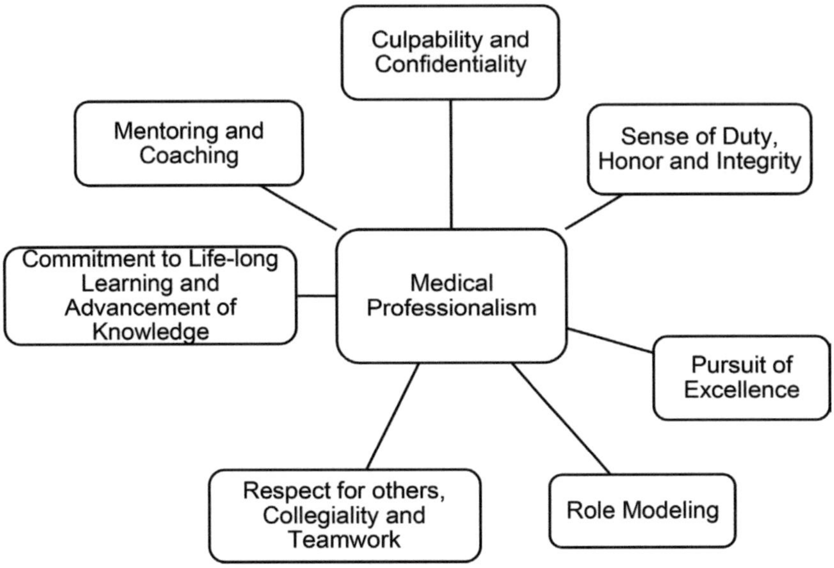

Figure 1.
The basic elements of medical professionalism [3].

to enhance patient satisfaction and improve the quality of healthcare services by fostering a deeper understanding of professionalism within healthcare institutions [9]. Consequently, healthcare institutions are obliged to develop continuous education programs and strategic plans to strengthen their understanding of professionalism. In this context, enhancing professionalism in healthcare services has the potential to positively impact both patient satisfaction and the quality of healthcare services. The enhancement of the professional ethos within healthcare institutions is a pivotal strategy for the augmentation of patient satisfaction and the refinement of healthcare services [10, 11]. In this regard, healthcare institutions should develop continuous education programs and strategic plans to strengthen their understanding of professionalism. This approach is expected to enhance patient satisfaction and improve the quality of healthcare services. The enhancement of professionalism is a pivotal factor in achieving sustainable success, as it leads to an increase in the effectiveness and quality of healthcare services, in addition to a concomitant rise in employee motivation. Consequently, cultivating a professional ethos within healthcare institutions is of paramount importance in enhancing patient satisfaction and reinforcing the motivation of healthcare professionals.

1.3 The relationship between professionalism and service quality

Professional behavior is closely related to factors that directly affect the patient experience, such as patient satisfaction and trust. Furthermore, the professional conduct of healthcare providers has been shown to enhance the quality of services throughout the hospital, as evidenced by improvements in clinical decision-making, ethical sensitivity, and team cohesion [12]. A plethora of studies have demonstrated that professional conduct exerts a favorable influence, especially on patient safety and employee motivation. It can thus be concluded that enhancing professionalism will contribute to sustainable success by increasing the effectiveness and quality of healthcare services, while also boosting employee motivation [13, 14]. The implementation of a professional approach within healthcare services has been demonstrated to enhance the effectiveness of such services.

Furthermore, the adoption of a professional approach has been shown to impact patient satisfaction, thereby positively strengthening employee motivation. In this context, the continuous enhancement of professionalism is a critical strategy for adapting to the complexity of the healthcare system and enhancing the effectiveness of multidisciplinary teams [15]. The enhancement of professionalism is a pivotal factor in achieving sustainable success, characterized by the improvement of healthcare service efficacy and quality, as well as the elevation of employee motivation. The concept of professionalism is an evolving one, and as such, it should be a continuous process of development. The enhancement of professionalism has been demonstrated to have a dual benefit; it has been shown to increase patient satisfaction in healthcare services and to strengthen employee motivation [16]. In this regard, enhancing professionalism can be identified as a pivotal strategy for the sustainable success of healthcare institutions. The role of professionalism in healthcare services has been demonstrated to have a dual impact on employee motivation and patient satisfaction.

1.4 Strategies to foster a culture of professionalism in healthcare

The creation and support of a culture of professionalism in healthcare institutions requires multi-level strategies that address individual behaviors, team dynamics, and organizational systems. At the individual level, the formation of a structured professional identity through ongoing education and reflective practice plays a pivotal role [17]. At the team level, the promotion of interprofessional collaboration and shared accountability has been demonstrated to be effective in establishing mutual trust and respect among healthcare professionals [18]. From an organizational perspective, leadership commitment is of great importance. It is incumbent upon managers to establish behavioral expectations, to serve as a model of professional conduct, and to incorporate professionalism into institutional policies and reward systems [19].

Furthermore, transparency and open communication—particularly in addressing medical errors—contribute to fostering a learning environment where professionalism is reinforced rather than undermined [20]. The integration of professionalism into human resource policies, mentorship programs, and evaluation systems is a crucial aspect of ensuring that professional values are not only encouraged but also systematically upheld across the organization. In this regard, professionalism becomes both a cultural norm and a strategic driver of high-quality healthcare delivery.

2. Conclusion

In conclusion, professionalism can be defined as a dynamic process that enhances the quality of healthcare services, improves patient satisfaction, and motivates employees. The development of professionalism within healthcare institutions requires a strategic approach that encompasses individual, team, and organizational levels. In this context, the concept of professionalism is closely tied to ethical values, individual responsibilities, organizational structures, and leadership approaches. The ongoing enhancement of professionalism is a pivotal strategy for adapting to the intricacies of the healthcare system and enhancing the efficacy of multidisciplinary teams. This process is conducive to sustainable success in healthcare delivery, engendering positive effects on both employee job satisfaction and patient outcomes.

Consequently, healthcare institutions must formulate strategic plans and implement ongoing education programs to enhance their understanding of professionalism, thereby optimizing the quality of healthcare services and improving patient satisfaction.

In conclusion, to accommodate the perpetual shifts in the realm of healthcare systems, there is an imperative for professionalism principles to be reinforced by a commitment to flexibility and innovation. The contemporary healthcare environment is characterized by several factors that are driving a shift in the concept of professionalism. These include the increasing prevalence of multidisciplinary work environments, the growing diversity of patients, and the ongoing digital transformation. This confluence of factors is prompting a re-evaluation of the very fabric of professionalism, leading to a more inclusive approach. Consequently, the concept of professionalism must be subject to continuous updating and development, both on an individual level, through the personal professional values of individuals, and on an institutional level, through the implementation of institutional strategies.

Author details

Hatice Esen Koc* and Nazife Öztürk
Antalya Training and Research Hospital, Antalya, Turkey

*Address all correspondence to: hatice.esen@gmail.com

References

[1] Chen M, Guan Q, Zhuang J. Patient-centered lean healthcare management from a humanistic perspective. BMC Health Services Research. 2024;**24**(1):2-15. DOI: 10.1186/s12913-024-11755-w

[2] Brennan MD, Monson V. Professionalism: Good for patients and health care organizations. Mayo Clinic Proceedings. 2014;**89**(5):644-652. DOI: 10.1016/j.mayocp.2014.01.011

[3] Bhardwaj A. Medical professionalism in the provision of clinical care in healthcare organizations. Journal of Healthcare Leadership. 2022;**14**(October):183-189. DOI: 10.2147/JHL.S383069

[4] Kaluc H, Kılıc SK, Kırılmaz S. A research aimed at the impact of strategic human resources management practices on turnover intention. Business & Management Studies: An International Journal. 2020;**8**(3):4069-4098. DOI: 10.15295/BMIJ.V8I5.1649

[5] Edgar A. Handbook of the philosophy of medicine. In: Handbook of the Philosophy of Medicine. Springer; 2017. pp. 1-21. DOI: 10.1007/978-94-017-8706-2

[6] Papadakis ND, Hodgson MA, Teherani CS, Kohatsu A. Unprofessional behaviour in medical school is associated with subsequent disciplinary action by a state medical board. Journal of Medical Licensure and Disipline. 2004;**9**(1):16-23. DOI: 10.30770/2572-1852-90.1.16

[7] Swick HM. Toward a normative definition of medical professionalism. Academic Medicine. 2000;**75**(6):612-616

[8] Cruess Y, Cruess RL, Steinert SR. Teaching Medical Professionalism: Supporting the Development of a Professional Identity. 2nd ed. Cambridge: Cambridge University Press; 2019

[9] Komsuoglu AF. Patient satisfaction and dental health service quality in private dental clinics. Journal of Statistic & Applied Sciences. 2022;**6**:1-11. DOI: 10.52693/jsas.1200905

[10] Ucanturk M. The importance of medical documentation and secretarial services in healthcare. In: Academic Research and Evaluations in the Field of Social Sciences-III -Sosyal Bilimler Alanında Akademik Araştırma Ve Değerlendirmeler-III. 2024. pp. 383-394. DOI: 10.58830/ozgur.pub604.c2710

[11] Semiz K, Semiz BB, Günes T. An investigation of measurement of perceived service quality and patient satisfaction in health. BMIJ. 2023;**11**(3):1130-1151. DOI: 10.15295/bmij.v11i3.2289 Araştırma

[12] Royal College of Physicians. Doctors in society: Medical professionalism in a changing world. In: Report of a Working Party of the Royal College of Physicians of London. London: RCP; 2005

[13] Patey AM, Fontaine G, Francis JJ, McCleary N, Presseau J, Grimshaw JM. Healthcare professional behaviour: Health impact, prevalence of evidence-based behaviours, correlates and interventions. Psychology & Health. 2023;**38**(6):766-794. DOI: 10.1080/08870446.2022.2100887

[14] Krijgsheld M, Tummers LG, Scheepers FE. Job performance in healthcare: A systematic review. BMC Health Services Research. 2022;**22**(1): 1-17. DOI: 10.1186/s12913-021-07357-5

[15] Blumenthal D. The vital role of professionalism in health care reform. Health Affair (Millwood). 1994;**13**(1):252-256. DOI: 10.1377/hlthaff.13.1.252

[16] Mason DJ. Professionalism in health care. The JAMA Forum. 2017;**317**(12):1023-1204. DOI: 10.1007/978-94-017-8688-1_30

[17] Cruess SR, Cruess RL, Steinert Y. Supporting the development of a professional identity: General principles. Medical Teacher. 2019;**41**(6):641-649. DOI: 10.1080/0142159X.2018.1536260

[18] Pechacek J, Anderson D, Lund R, Drill-Mellum L. Healthy work environments: An interprofessional partnership model to promote positive workplace culture. Interdisciplinary Journal of Partnership Studies. 2022;**9**(2):7. DOI: 10.24926/ijps.v9i2.4978

[19] Jovanovski N, Jaeger T. Demystifying 'diet culture': Exploring the meaning of diet culture in online 'anti-diet' feminist, fat activist, and health professional communities. Womens Student Int Forum. 2022;**90**:102558. DOI: 10.1016/j.wsif.2021.102558

[20] Desai MK, Kapadia JD. Medical professionalism and ethics. Journal of Pharmacology and Pharmacotherapeutics. 2022;**13**(2):113-118. DOI: 10.1177/0976500X221111448

Chapter 3

Perioperative Care, Operating Room Efficiency, and Surgical Outcome Improvement

Matthew Mazurek

Abstract

Perioperative care spans preoperative preparation, intraoperative management, and postoperative recovery, with the overarching goal of optimizing safety, outcomes, efficiency, and quality. Beyond cost reduction and institutional performance, high-functioning perioperative systems elevate the patient experience. Interventions such as streamlined scheduling and enhanced recovery after surgery (ERAS) protocols, supported by interdisciplinary collaboration, have reduced surgical delays, hospital length of stay, and readmissions. Advances in anesthetic techniques and monitoring further promote safety by lowering surgical site infection risk, minimizing anesthesia-related morbidity, and enhancing comfort during recovery. A patient-centered model, including preoperative clinics for risk stratification, comorbidity management, and patient engagement, aligns surgical success with functional recovery and improved quality of life. Operational strategies using lean and six sigma methodologies, coupled with performance metrics such as on-time starts and turnover time, strengthen efficiency, satisfaction, and financial sustainability. Yet, without a supportive work culture, such initiatives often falter. Building trust, teamwork, and engagement fosters a positive environment where improvement efforts in clinical pathways, operations, and culture can succeed. Ultimately, aligning efficiency with safety allows perioperative care to achieve its core mission: delivering high-quality, patient-centered surgical outcomes while ensuring healthcare system sustainability.

Keywords: perioperative care, enhanced recovery after surgery (ERAS), patient-centered outcomes, operational efficiency, healthcare sustainability

1. Introduction

Peri-operative care of surgical patients has evolved and changed dramatically in the last two decades. There is a new appreciation that a patient is on a surgical 'journey' throughout the perioperative period of care. The three phases of surgical care, including preoperative, operative, and postoperative are linked and each phase can negatively or positively impact patient outcomes. Economic pressures in the healthcare industry are forcing hospitals to focus efforts on efficient operating room throughput and operations as well. Improving clinical care and focusing on efficient operations management requires an interdisciplinary approach, and it can be challenging for healthcare organizations to successfully initiate change. Current clinical and operational strategies offer practical solutions for healthcare organizations and leaders to create and maintain improved surgical care outcomes using resources more efficiently.

1.1 Perioperative surgical home (PSH) model

How can healthcare organizations address common and costly operating room (OR) efficiency gaps? What strategies can be applied to design a patient workflow environment for increased efficiency, safety, and patient and provider satisfaction? Increasing cost and non-optimal patient outcomes are driving new models for the provision of surgical care. Payers and health insurers are moving from paying for services separately to 'bundled payment' arrangements. Through a 'bundled payment,' the payers provide a lump sum payment that includes all services provided for a surgical patient, including surgical fees, facility fees, anesthesia services fees, and post-operative care and follow-up. These novel payment arrangements have compelled health systems and providers to reduce expenses and perioperative complications [1].

The PSH model is a novel and innovative approach for the care of surgical patients incorporating, a longitudinal, interdisciplinary umbrella of services led by a coordinated care team [2]. The PSH uses a patient-centered approach, and the episode of care begins the time a patient is scheduled for surgery until the patient fully recovers from surgery. Each step along this continuum of care is critical to the success and outcome of the next phase of care. As previously stated, care of a surgical patient occurs in three distinct phases: preoperative, intraoperative, and post-operative (**Figure 1**). Each phase requires completion of specific tasks to prepare the patient for the next phase of the surgical journey.

Recent research has demonstrated that the PSH model is effective at reducing costs associated with care, increasing OR efficiency, and reducing same day cancelation rates of surgical procedures [2]. Similar to other industries, quality and outcomes are improved with standardized processes and approaches. Processes for patient care can be standardized, but the complex nature of illness and other mitigating factors,

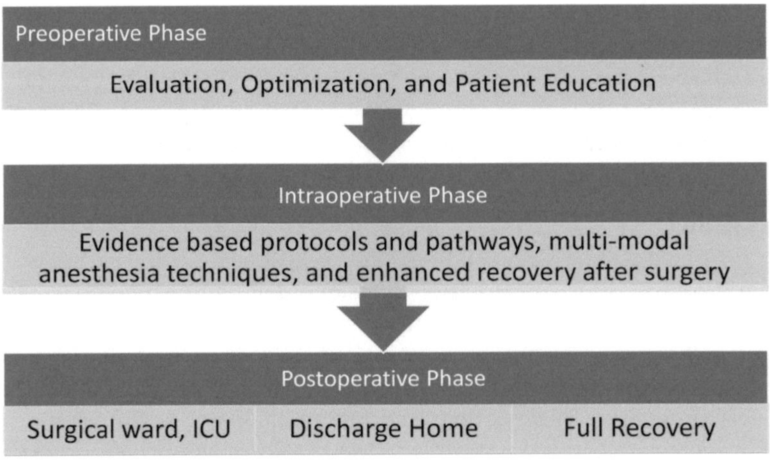

Figure 1.
Perioperative surgical home care pathway.

including the surgical skill of the surgeon, can influence outcome variability, complication rates, and associated increases in cost [3–5]. Anesthetic techniques have evolved to reduce the intra- and post-operative use of opioids, and this reduces the length of time required to recover from surgery.

1.2 Preoperative phase strategies

Once the patient is scheduled for surgery, the patient must be evaluated as a candidate for the surgical procedure. Many patients presenting for surgery are medically complex with multiple comorbidities, and same day cancelation of a surgical procedure is often the result of inadequate patient preparation or untreated medical conditions. A canceled surgical procedure results in lost revenue, an increase in operating room expenses as the labor cost is absorbed, and a frustrated and dissatisfied patient. To reduce the number of case cancelations and prepare patients for surgery, preoperative clinics have emerged as a solution [6].

Preoperative clinics have two major functions: patient preparation and education. Several models of the preoperative clinic are utilized depending on resources and demand. Many clinics are led by an anesthesiologist and a team comprised of nurses or, more recently, nurse practitioners and physician assistants. Other models solely employ nurses or nurse practitioners. Non-anesthesiologists can also lead a clinic team or evaluate patients, but these individuals must be trained to perform a thorough preoperative evaluation.

Not all patients require a specific preoperative evaluation. Younger, healthier patients requiring less complicated or routine procedures, for example, do not need extensive workups and interventions. For these patients, a telephone call or brief telehealth visit often suffices. If it is determined that the patient requires further diagnostic testing or treatment, the patient can be scheduled for a formal appointment in the clinic.

In addition to patient preparation for surgery, other critical tasks include obtaining prior authorization and approval for the procedure and ensuring special equipment or resources are available for the procedure. A practical approach is the use of a preoperative checklist the day prior to surgery (**Table 1**). A daily huddle with preoperative, OR, and postoperative nurses and managers can identify which components of the checklist are missing. This process reduces surgery cancelations and delays.

A preoperative clinic and completion of other tasks do increase the cost of preoperative care, and a recent study found that costs can be up to 45% higher [7]. Despite this increase in cost, there is overall cost reduction through fewer complications, delays, and a shorter length-of-stay (LOS) [7]. Healthcare systems may be reluctant to invest in the preoperative preparation of patients, but if overall costs are reduced, there is significant return on the investment.

Case scheduled with OR start time and anticipated length of surgery	Yes	No
History, physical and consent complete	Yes	No
Prior authorization approved	Yes	No
Special equipment, resources, and medical device representatives available	Yes	No
Patient education and phone call for arrival time and other instructions	Yes	No
Disposition (admit to floor, ICU, etc.) or discharge home	Yes	No

Table 1.
Preoperative checklist day prior to scheduled surgery or procedure.

1.3 Intraoperative phase strategies

In 1994, Engelman and other colleagues published a paper on the results of 'fast-tracking' patients undergoing coronary artery bypass surgery. Their goal was to reduce extubation time post-surgery. They successfully fast-tracked patients and the time to extubation decreased from 22 hours to 15 hours. In turn, this reduced the LOS in the ICU by 21% and there was an overall 19% reduction in the hospital LOS. LOS directly impacts resource costs for surgical procedures. Fast-tracking patients was the first initiative that led to the creation of enhanced recovery after surgery (ERAS) protocols [8].

Enhanced recovery after surgery protocols are clinical pathways of care for surgical patients incorporating principles of the PSH. ERAS protocols, however, provide specific operative day clinical care pathways for patients. The main goals of ERAS protocols are decreased complications, improved postoperative pain management, reduced length of stay, and faster recovery after surgery. These protocols produce better outcomes, and there is a significant reduction in overall cost for care [7, 9]. In the past decade, the number of different ERAS protocols has expanded to include nearly all types of surgery, including total joint replacements, urological and gynecological procedures, and colorectal procedures.

1.4 Postoperative phase strategies

The postoperative phase is just as important as the other two phases. It is a mistake not to invest resources and effort in patient recovery. During this phase, avoiding postoperative complications is essential, as this increases morbidity and mortality. ERAS protocols reduce LOS, and for patients who are being discharged the same day, ensuring adequate postoperative care is available is critical. Patients also desire a recovery that is as comfortable as possible with a return to normal or improved function as soon as possible [7].

The social determinants of health impact all phases of surgical care, and for patients without resources or support, the recovery journey is more difficult. Research has shown that patients with lower incomes, lower health literacy, and lower social support take longer to recover and are at increased risk of developing complications. Engaging with social workers, community programs, and partnerships, and educating surgeons and other care team members can help reduce complications [10].

It is important to appreciate that the clinical care pathway occurs within a larger ecosystem and environment of care that is complex. Operational efficiency is just as important as the clinical care pathway. Efficient systems imbue quality and safety, encourage staff engagement, and create positive loops for continual improvement.

1.5 Operating room efficiency

Intraoperative care is the most expensive and resource-intensive phase in perioperative care. Operating rooms are the financial nexus of a hospital and account for up to 40% of a hospital's costs and 60–70% of hospital revenues [11, 12]. Maximizing efficiency maximizes the revenue stream for the hospital and leads to secondary benefits, including increased OR throughput, patient safety, and increased patient and surgeon satisfaction.

Instead of exploring what drives OR efficiency, it is more useful to explore and address what drives OR *inefficiency*. Identifying factors, processes, or lack of resources that produce bottlenecks, delays in care, or errors is the first step in creating a more efficient operating room environment. Current financial pressures have catapulted this issue into the spotlight in many healthcare organizations.

1.6 Identifying causes for operating room inefficiency

Any process depending on inputs and outputs in a complex environment is exposed to bottlenecks, delays, and quality output errors. Identifying the causes is challenging and time-consuming. On any given operative day, the OR inputs (patients and resources for surgery) are prepared for surgery before the patient enters the room. Once in the room, the patient is anesthetized, positioned, and surgery commences.

Surgeons vary in their skills, speed, and efficiency. Some surgeons can perform a routine knee replacement in under 1 hour, while others perform the same procedure in 2 to 3 hours. Obviously, in an eight-hour OR day, the faster surgeon can complete more cases than the slower surgeon. Therefore, scheduling OR time for the surgeons must account for the difference in time each performs the surgery. Scheduling by case type can create problems for the daily OR schedule. For example, if the 'median' time for a knee replacement is used, the slower surgeon will be 'over-booked' and the faster surgeon will be 'under-booked.'

Surgeon A (slower): Case Length Average is 135 minutes.

Surgeon B (faster): Case Length Average is 56 minutes.

The overall average is (135 minutes +56 minutes)/2 = 95.5 minutes.

Operating room scheduling, also known as 'block-time' allotment, should reflect and account for the average time it takes for that surgeon to complete a certain type of procedure. Environments that do not account for this are particularly prone to inefficient use of labor. Idle ORs and overtime create lost opportunity costs and increases in overall labor costs. Additionally, patient satisfaction is impacted by delays, and staff are often pressured to perform tasks more quickly if the OR is behind schedule. A time-pressured, stressed staff creates an environment that is prone to producing errors, which increase complication rates and patient harm.

1.7 Little's law

As previously stated, operative care occurs within a system process. Patients arrive for surgery in the pre-operative area and are transported to the OR for a procedure. Upon completion of the procedure, the patients are transported to a post-operative recovery unit (PACU) for further care. Essentially, patients are in a 'line' or a 'queue' as they arrive on the operative day.

John Little, a physicist at Massachusetts Institute of Technology, developed a theorem known as *Little's Law* that relates the average number of items in a system (L) to the average arrival rate (λ) multiplied by the average time an item spends in the system (W). The more items in process, the longer it takes for each of them to be completed [13]. If two of the variables are known, the missing variable can be calculated using the formula for Little's Law:

$$L = \lambda W$$

Within the context of the OR, **L** is the number of patients waiting or actively undergoing procedures. **λ** is the number of completed surgeries per unit of time, and **W** is the average time a patient spends within the OR system.

As an example, an OR suite performs an average of 20 surgeries per day (throughput). If the average flow time for a patient, from entering the pre-op area to being discharged from the PACU, is 6 hours (0.25 days), then, according to Little's Law:

$$L\ (\text{Inventory}) = 20\ \text{surgeries/day} * 0.25\ \text{days/surgery} = 5\ \text{patients}$$

This means, on average, there will be five patients in various stages of the surgical process within the OR suite at any given time. Reducing the average number of patients waiting or in process (inventory) can be accomplished through increasing the throughput (performing more surgeries per day) or reducing the flow time (improving efficiency, for example, by streamlining OR turnover times).

Little's Law is simple and powerful, and understanding the relationships between these variables can provide the data for process improvement. Areas for improvement include optimal staffing and capacity planning, identifying bottlenecks, improving patient flow and reducing wait times, and assessing the impact of changes.

Accurately measuring the time a patient spends in each phase of the operative day is necessary for process improvement. The steps involved in each phase of care are as follows:

$$\text{Arrival and registration} \rightarrow \text{Preparation} \rightarrow \text{Time in OR} \rightarrow \text{PACU} \rightarrow \text{Admit to floor or Discharge home.}$$

In parallel, there is preparation of the operating room and turnover time between each case:

$$\text{Instrument sterilization and preparation} \rightarrow \text{OR setup time} \rightarrow \text{Surgery} \rightarrow \text{Turnover time [TOT] (time to prepare for next procedure).}$$

One of the advantages of the electronic medical record system is the time-stamping feature for most tasks. As an example, circulating nurses document a patient's arrival to the OR, and the anesthesia providers document when a patient is intubated and ready for surgery. Time stamped data, if done accurately, can be used to identify bottlenecks and opportunities for improvement.

Once a bottleneck or source of delay has been identified, a *Fishbone Diagram* can help identify causes [14]. For example, most operating rooms have a scheduled start time of 7:30 AM. A first case on-time (FCOT) start is critical, as delays impact subsequent procedure start times for that room. There are a cascading and snowballing effect. A Fishbone Diagram for the first case on-time start (FCOT) delays is shown in **Figure 2**. Reasons for delays are presented in a qualitative manner.

Once delays have been identified, the most common cause for FCOT delay can be addressed through a change initiative. If the OR is not ready, for example, a focus group can be created to identify whether it is a workflow problem, a personnel problem, or a lack of equipment, etc. Another frequent problem is surgeon or anesthesia providers arriving too late to start a case. For example, if a surgeon consistently arrives at 7:25 AM for a 7:30 AM start, it is impossible for the surgeon to address all concerns, answer questions, and complete other tasks before the procedure. This is a professionalism issue and will be discussed in a separate section.

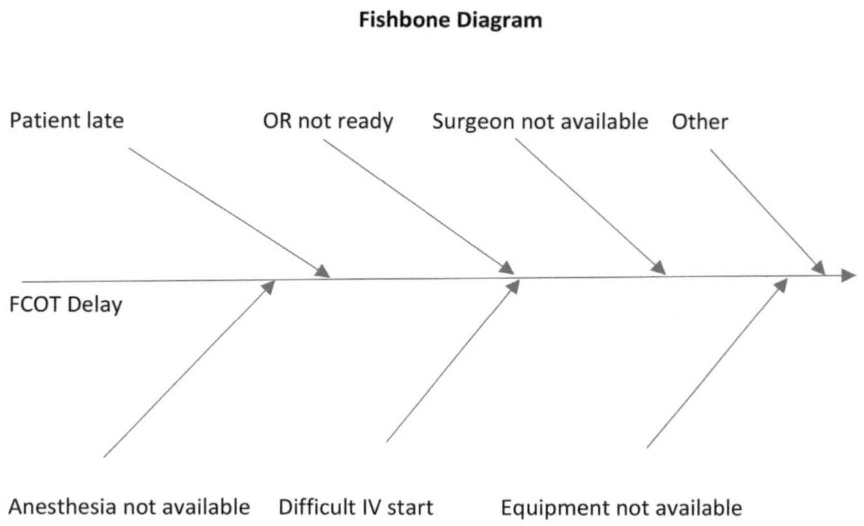

Figure 2.
Fishbone diagram and reasons for FCOT delay.

1.8 Strategies for implementing a more efficient operating room

Implementing change in healthcare is challenging. There are numerous parallel tasks from different departments interdependent on other departments, and effective leadership is essential for change and continued success. There are strategies for implementing change, and utilizing the same approach as other businesses in different sectors has demonstrated successful change efforts.

1.9 Models for change management in the perioperative setting

The healthcare environment in general is changing rapidly. As previously discussed, new payment models, an emphasis on quality and outcomes, and now, adopting artificial intelligence (AI) have placed pressure on healthcare organizations to respond and implement changes. Agile, open, and adaptable systems are more successful. Appreciating that change is a process that is never fully completed sets the tone for continuous improvement. Extensive efforts, education, and training around change management have not prevented failure. The complexity of the environment and lack of consistent approaches are contributing factors.

The most commonly applied change management models in healthcare are Lewin's Model and Kotter's 8-Step Model. Kurt Lewin introduced his model in the 1940s. The approach begins with 'unfreezing' a process and examining inefficiencies. Changes are made to the process after analysis, and the process is 'refrozen' and incorporated into a new workflow. This three-step model has become one of the most widely used approaches for organizational change, but critics have argued that the approach is too simple, linear, prescriptive, and does not account for the complexity of modern businesses and other organizations. Despite the limitations of this model, it has been used in simpler processes that are linear in nature with fewer input variables. The OR, for example, is a perfect example of an environment where patients go through a series of processes that are standardized and predictable [15–17].

One of the most influential variables impacting the success of any process change is effective leadership, and in healthcare, clinician engagement is critical. Kotter's 8-step model is a modern approach and factors in the complexity of modern organizational processes [15]. Additionally, the model appreciates the impact and importance of effective leadership. Kotter's eight steps are as follows:

1. Create of Sense of Urgency: Motivating key stakeholders on the reasons for change includes effectively communicating the need for change.

2. Building a Coalition: At its core, change management is a group effort. This stage includes forming a group of influential individuals who are engaged and believe in the necessary change.

3. Develop a Vision and Strategy: Create a clear vision and develop a strategy to achieve the vision.

4. Communicate the Vision: Sharing the vision with all stakeholders and those impacted by the change is critical to gain support.

5. Empower Employees for Action: Engaging those directly impacted by change and removing barriers for employees.

6. Generate Short-Term Wins: Building and maintaining momentum is achieved through acknowledging the success of short-term goals.

7. Consolidate gains and Produce More Change: Use the successes of smaller change to drive further change.

8. Anchor New Change: Ensure changes are implemented and integrated into the organization's culture for sustainability.

Two recent studies using Kotter's 8-Step Model demonstrated the success of a quality improvement project in an ear, nose, and throat (ENT) surgical department in an academic department in Canada. Sustained high clinical performance was achieved through the program compared to patients on a non-structured clinical pathway. Another project reduced surgical site infections from breast surgeries from 7–2% and readmission rates from infection from 2.2–0% [15]. These remarkable results did not increase overall surgical cost or rely on increased use of resources. Recent developments in artificial intelligence, regulatory compliance, financial pressures, and short-staffed environments have made the last phase, anchoring, increasingly difficult. There is a lot of disruption, both external and internal, in healthcare delivery, and adapting to the changing environment quickly requires more rapid, agile responses.

1.10 Employing lean six sigma strategies

Lean and Six Sigma strategies are process improvement tools using objective data and key performance indicators for process improvement. Kotter's 8-step approach incorporates the human factors of communication, strategy formulation, and relationship and team building efforts to effect change. Lean and Six Sigma are specific tools, and their utility in the perioperative period is extremely valuable as it is iterative

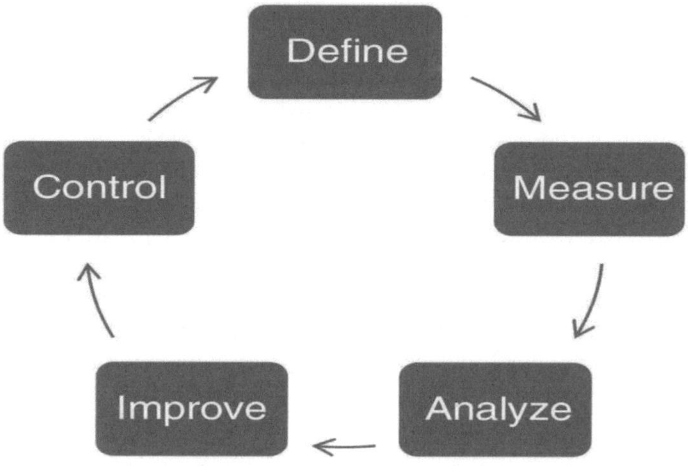

Figure 3.
DMAIC cycle.

and examine processes in more detail. Unlike 'anchoring' change, it uses data to make further changes and improvements using the define, measure, analyze, improve, and control (DMAIC) methodology (**Figure 3**) [18].

The first step is defining the boundaries for the process being analyzed. In the OR, for example, FCOTs are defined through the time a patient enters the OR. As an example, if a patient enters the OR after 07:30 AM, it is a failure to start on time. The second step is measuring and analyzing the data. Continuing with the example, what specifically caused the delay (common reasons are lack of equipment, providers arrive late, patient arrives late, etc.)? Once the data has been processed, categories of factors can be charted and analyzed. Once processes are analyzed, efforts to improve the process can be implemented. During the control phase, the process is continually measured to ensure it does not degrade. In this iterative cycle, continual improvement is possible.

1.11 TeamSTEPPS

In 2006, the Agency for Healthcare Research and Quality (AHRQ) and the United States Department of Defense (US DoD) produced an evidence-based resource for team training in healthcare. The resource, Team Strategies and Tools to Enhance Performance and Patient Safety (TeamSTEPPS), adopts a crew resource management tool created by the United States Department of Defense for the operating room and perioperative setting. Using briefings and huddles, TeamSTEPPS encourages situational awareness and communication. Central to the training for TeamSTEPPS are four competencies in the domains of leadership, situational monitoring, mutual support, and communication [19].

Numerous studies have demonstrated the effectiveness of using TeamSTEPPS in the clinical environment in reducing errors and increasing efficiency [20]. Healthcare organizations utilizing this approach improve and enhance employee and staff perceptions of teamwork and patient safety. Because this approach incorporates clinical and operational components for care, it is an amalgamation that can have a positive impact on creating a positive cultural environment.

1.12 Cultural influences and change management: Building trust and safety

Peter Drucker, noted management expert, author, and professor, famously stated, "Culture eats strategy for breakfast." Change initiatives fail when there is a lack of trust, transparency, and engagement. The complexity of the OR environment creates tension and stress in a high acuity environment. And the 'assembly line' process is ripe for conflict if there are issues and concerns with delays, errors, or other inefficient processes that lead to frustration and finger-pointing at other team members.

Personal interactions and how staff communicate either foster a respectful environment or create tension, conflict, and stress. The current focus on the influence of positive culture is the result of ongoing efforts to increase safety and reduce errors that harm patients. A poor cultural environment impacts patient care and outcomes.

There are four core elements of perioperative culture: trust, respect, communication, and purpose. The core elements are the foundation for a good working environment and also serve as a springboard for change. Unlike many other industries, the OR is a unique environment where critical tasks occur in an 'open environment' that relies on communication between all parties. Perioperative safety depends on open, accurate, and timely communication. An environment of fear and distrust disrupts communication chains, and the performance of all individuals suffers in a tense, disruptive environment [21–23].

Respectful environments produce better teams, and instead of blaming individuals for errors, more modern approaches include huddles when errors occur, so they can be prevented. Errors are often system-based or communication-based. The OR environment, similar to the airline industry, performs better with checklists and closed communication loops. The universal 'time out' protocol was developed to help prevent wrong-site surgery and other avoidable errors. It works, but it depends on a culture of safety and trust. Successful change depends on sharing a vision and strategy with a positive culture.

1.13 Professionalism and behavior management strategies

Disruptive behaviors directly impact patient care. The Joint Commission, recognizing the impact of disruptive behaviors on patient care, published *Sentinel Event Alert 40* in 2008 [24]. Historically, the operating room environment has had a poor reputation for tolerating unacceptable behaviors. Since the publication of the Joint Commission's Alert, healthcare systems have created and adopted professional conduct policies and committees to address concerns.

A just, safe culture depends on healthcare leadership enforcing professional conduct policies objectively and fairly, regardless of the status or role of the attributed individual. Treating staff with a double standard and inconsistently enforcing policy erodes trust and creates a negative and toxic culture. For example, if a surgeon arrives late on a daily basis for scheduled cases and the issue is not addressed at the same time staff is disciplined for similar behaviors, the perception is that the surgeon's behavior is tolerated because the surgeon creates the revenue for the operating room.

2. Conclusion

Delivering high-quality, safe, efficient perioperative care is possible when efforts to improve clinical and operational pathways in a positive cultural environment are

DOI: http://dx.doi.org/10.5772/intechopen.1013704

prioritized. Healthcare organizations and leaders must understand that these processes are inextricably intertwined and interdependent. Focus groups and specialized committees creating programs, initiatives, and protocols create accountability and shared responsibility. Clinical staff, including physicians, nurses, pharmacists, techs, and other stakeholders, offer perspectives on workflow and culture not fully appreciated by non-clinical leaders and administrators. Clinical pathways and operation management strategies continue to evolve, especially as new medical knowledge is gleaned from research on improving the perioperative patient journey.

Author details

Matthew Mazurek
Department of Anesthesiology, Yale University School of Medicine, New Haven, Connecticut, United States

*Address all correspondence to: matthew.mazurek@yale.edu

References

[1] Dessebe O, Lanz T, Kain Z, Cannesson M. The perioperative surgical home: An innovative, patient-centered and cost-effective perioperative care model. Anaesthesia Critical Care & Pain Medicine. 2016;**35**(1):59-66. DOI: 10.1016/j.accpm.2015.08.001

[2] Cline K, Clement V, Rock-Klotz Kash B, Steel C, Miller T. Improving the cost, quality, and safety of perioperative care: A systematic review of the literature on implementation of the perioperative surgical home. Journal of Clinical Anesthesia. 2020;**63**:109760. DOI: 10.1016./j.jclinane.2020.109760

[3] Lyman W et al. The next step in surgical quality improvement: Outcome situational awareness. Canadian Journal of Surgery. 2020;**63**(2):E120-E122

[4] Amati M, Valnegri A, Bressan A, La Regina D, Tassone C, Lo PA, et al. Reducing changeover time between surgeries through lean thinking: An action research project. Frontiers in Medicine. 2022;**9**(822964)

[5] Mazurek Matt J. Improving operations, from Preop to postop. Journal of Healthcare Management. 2024;**69**(1):8-11. DOI: 10.1097/JHM-D-23-00238

[6] Meyers N, Giron S, Burkard J, Bush R. Preventing surgical delay and cancellation with patient-centered interventions. Journal of PeriAnesthesia Nursing. 2021;**36**:334-338

[7] Bertocci E et al. Cost saving analysis of an enhanced recovery after surgery (ERAS) program for elective colorectal surgery in an ERAS qualified and training center. World Journal of Surgery. 2025;**49**:850-858. DOI: 10.1002/wjs/12548

[8] Engelman R, Rousou J, Flack J. Fast-track recovery of the coronary artery bypass patient. Annals of Thoracic Surgery. 1994;**58**:1742-1746

[9] Echeverria-Villalobos M, Stoicea N. Enhance recovery after surgery (ERAS): A perspective review postoperative pain management under ERAS pathways and its role on opioid crisis in the United States. Clinical Journal of Pain. 2020; **36**(3):219-226. DOI: 10.1097/AJP.0000000000000792

[10] Devin C, Shaffer V. Social determinants of health and impact in the perioperative space. Clinics in Colon and Rectal Surgery. 2023;**36**(3):206-209. DOI: 10.1055/s-0043-1761155

[11] Healey T, El-Othmani M, Healey J, Peterson T, Saleh K. Improving operating room efficiency, part 1: General managerial and preoperative strategies. Journal of Bone and Joint Surgical Review. 2015;**3**(10):1-10

[12] Rothstein D, Raval M. Operating room efficiency. Seminars in Pediatric Surgery. 2018;**27**(2):79-85. DOI: 10.1053/j.sempedsurg.2018.02.044

[13] Kim S, Whitt W. Estimating waiting times with the time-varying Little's law. Probability in the Engineering Informational Sciences. 2013;**27**:471-506

[14] Kumah A, Nwogu CN, Issah AR, Obot E, Kanamitie DT, Sifa JS, et al. Cause-and-effect (fishbone) diagram: A tool for generating and organizing quality improvement ideas. Global Journal of Quality and Safety in Healthcare. 2024;**7**(2):85-87. DOI: 10.36401/JQSH-23-42

[15] Harrison R et al. Where do models for change management, improvement

and implementation meet? A systematic review of the applications of change management models in healthcare. Journal of Healthcare Leadership. 2021; **13**:85-108

[16] Hastings B. Guidance for successful healthcare transformation: A systematic review of change management practices and outcomes. Australian Journal of Management. 2025;**50**(3):985-1005. DOI: 10.177/03128962241307347

[17] Burnes B. The origin's of Lewin's three-step model of change. The Journal of Applied Behavioral Science. 2020; **56**(1):32-59. DOI: 10.177/0021886319892685

[18] Pérez-Balboa IC, Caballero-Morales SO. Define, measure, analyze, improve, control (DMAIC). In: García Alcaraz JL, Robles GC, Realyvásquez Vargas A, editors. Lean Manufacturing in Latin America. Cham: Springer; 2025. DOI: 10.1007/978-3-031-70984-5_15

[19] Weld L et al. TeamSTEPPS improves operating room efficiency and patient safety. American Journal of Medical Quality. 2016;**31**(5):408-414. DOI: 10.177/1062860615583671

[20] Shi Y et al. TeamSTEPPS improves patient safety. BMJ Open Quality. 2024; **13**:e002669. DOI: 10.1136/bmjoq-2023-002669

[21] Bello C. Building a well-balanced culture in the perioperative setting. Best Practice & Research Clinical Anaesthesiology. 2022;**36**:247-256. DOI: 10.1016/j.bpa.2022.05.003

[22] Hussain S et al. Kurt Lewin's change model: A critical review of the role of leadership and employee involvement in organizational change. Journal of Innovation & Knowledge. 2018;**3**: 123-127. DOI: 10.1016/j.jik.2016.07.002

[23] Hughes M. Leading changes: Why transformation explanations fail. Leadership. 2016;**12**(4):449-469. DOI: 10.1177/1742715015571393

[24] Joint Commission. Behaviors that undermine a culture of safety. Sentinel Event Alert. 2008;**40**(40)

Chapter 4

Hospital Efficiency and Patient Recovery: The Impact of Enhanced Recovery after Surgery (ERAS) Protocols on Healthcare Quality

Ömer Faruk Sağlam

Abstract

Enhanced recovery after surgery (ERAS) protocols represent a paradigm shift in perioperative care, designed to minimize surgical stress, accelerate recovery, and improve outcomes through standardized, evidence-based practices. Originating in colorectal surgery, ERAS has since been successfully adapted across numerous specialties, demonstrating consistent reductions in complication rates, hospital length of stay, and opioid use. From a hospital management perspective, ERAS not only enhances clinical quality but also improves operational efficiency by increasing bed turnover, reducing costs, and standardizing care workflows. Successful implementation requires a multidisciplinary approach, robust leadership, staff education, patient engagement, and data-driven quality improvement. Despite challenges such as cultural resistance, logistical constraints, and the need for sustained compliance, ERAS protocols have proven adaptable and beneficial across diverse healthcare systems. Ultimately, ERAS delivers a high-value care model that aligns patient-centered outcomes with institutional performance goals, making it a strategic priority for hospitals aiming to elevate surgical quality and efficiency.

Keywords: enhanced recovery after surgery (ERAS), postoperative care, hospital administration, surgical recovery, clinical pathways

1. Introduction

Enhanced recovery after surgery (ERAS) is an evidence-based paradigm shift in perioperative care designed to minimize surgical stress and accelerate recovery. First conceptualized in the 1990s by Henrik Kehlet in Denmark, early ERAS efforts demonstrated remarkable outcomes—for example, patients undergoing major colorectal surgery could be discharged in about 2 days postoperatively instead of the traditional 10 days [1]. Originally developed in Northern Europe for colorectal procedures, ERAS programs have since been adopted globally and expanded across multiple surgical disciplines, including orthopedic, thoracic, gynecologic, urologic, and others [1]. ERAS pathways are multidisciplinary, patient-centered care protocols spanning the preoperative, intraoperative, and postoperative phases. By implementing numerous evidence-based interventions in concert, ERAS aims to reduce the physiological stress of surgery, thereby improving patient outcomes and speeding up recovery [2, 3]. Over the past decades, this approach has transformed perioperative care and has become an indispensable standard in many surgical fields, marking a new era of improved surgical quality and efficiency [4, 5].

From a hospital management perspective, ERAS protocols offer not only clinical benefits but also operational advantages. Studies consistently report that ERAS improves key outcomes such as complication rates, length of hospital stay, and patient satisfaction, while simultaneously lowering healthcare costs [1, 6–8]. This dual impact on patient recovery and hospital efficiency makes ERAS an appealing strategy for healthcare administrators seeking to enhance the quality of care and optimize resource utilization. The following sections provide a comprehensive overview of ERAS protocols—their core components, effects on patient recovery across various specialties, and implications for hospital efficiency—and discuss strategies for successful implementation along with common challenges from an administrative viewpoint.

2. Core components of ERAS protocols

ERAS protocols are built on a foundation of multiple interdependent interventions that span the entire surgical journey. These core components can be categorized into preoperative, intraoperative, and postoperative measures, all aiming to standardize care and reduce variability from admission through recovery [5, 6, 8, 9]. By adhering to these elements, hospitals seek to attenuate the stress response to surgery, optimize physiological function, and facilitate faster recovery.

2.1 Preoperative optimization and education

Before surgery, ERAS emphasizes thorough patient evaluation and optimization of health status. This includes nutritional assessment and supplementation (if needed), encouraging smoking cessation and alcohol moderation, and managing chronic conditions ahead of time [1]. Patient and family education is a cornerstone—patients are counseled on what to expect and actively engaged in their care plan. Unlike traditional approaches that mandated prolonged fasting, ERAS protocols allow minimal fasting: clear fluids (and often a carbohydrate-rich drink) up to 2 hours before anesthesia, rather than overnight, to reduce dehydration and insulin resistance [8, 9]. Bowel preparation is avoided or minimized when possible to prevent undue discomfort and electrolyte disturbances [10]. Overall, the preoperative phase in ERAS sets the stage for a smoother surgical course by ensuring patients are in the best possible condition and fully informed participants in their care.

2.2 Intraoperative strategies

During surgery, ERAS protocols promote techniques that minimize tissue trauma and maintain homeostasis. Whenever feasible, minimally invasive surgery (MIS) techniques (laparoscopy or robotic surgery) are preferred, as they are associated with less pain and quicker recovery [1]. Anesthesia management is tailored for rapid recovery: this includes avoidance of long-acting sedatives, use of short-acting anesthetic agents, and multimodal analgesia to reduce opioid use (e.g., regional blocks, epidurals, and non-opioid analgesics are employed) [11]. Optimal fluid management is another key element—goal-directed fluid therapy to avoid both fluid overload and deficit, helping to maintain perfusion without causing edema [1]. Intraoperative warming is standard to prevent hypothermia, which is linked to increased complications. Prophylaxis for nausea/vomiting (PONV) is given to enable early oral intake, and antibiotics are used appropriately to prevent infections. Additionally, surgeons aim to reduce the use of tubes and drains unless absolutely indicated [5]. Each of these intraoperative practices is evidence-based and contributes to less physiological derangement, enabling patients to emerge from surgery in a more stable state conducive to fast-track recovery [1, 10].

2.3 Postoperative rehabilitation

The postoperative phase in ERAS is geared toward early recovery of function. Early mobilization is a hallmark—patients are encouraged to get out of bed and start walking within hours of surgery, rather than days [11]. Early ambulation helps prevent complications such as deep vein thrombosis, pneumonia, and muscle deconditioning; studies in colorectal surgery show that even a few hours' difference in mobilization can shorten hospital stay by 1.5–3 days on average [11]. Similar benefits of early mobilization have been observed in orthopedic surgery, with one study noting a ~1.9-day reduction in length of stay for total hip and knee replacement patients who walked soon after surgery [11]. Along with mobilization, early oral nutrition is promoted—patients resume a normal diet as early as the day of surgery or the next morning, avoiding the traditional prolonged fasting until bowel function returns [1, 2, 9]. Tolerating a diet earlier contributes to quicker recovery of gastrointestinal function and energy. Postoperative analgesia under ERAS is managed *via* multimodal pain control, continuing the intraoperative plan: by combining non-opioid analgesics, regional anesthesia techniques, and sparing use of opioids, patients experience adequate pain relief with fewer opioid-related side effects (respiratory depression, nausea, and ileus) [11]. This approach has been shown to not only improve pain scores but also facilitate faster mobilization and reduce hospital length of stay [11]. Other ERAS elements include early removal of catheters and IVs, nausea control, and daily activity goals.

Collectively, these core components form a cohesive pathway. The success of ERAS lies in its holistic approach, addressing nutrition, analgesia, mobility, and other factors simultaneously [11]. Significant gains stem from the cumulative effect of small improvements rather than any single intervention. ERAS protocols are regularly updated as new evidence emerges to optimize outcomes [5]. Hospitals implementing ERAS often adopt standardized order sets or checklists reflecting these components to ensure high protocol compliance and consistency of care.

3. Effects on patient recovery across surgical specialties

A key strength of ERAS is its broad applicability, with principles initially developed for colorectal surgery now benefiting many other specialties [12, 13]. By reducing surgical stress and standardizing care, ERAS improves recovery metrics like complications, hospital stay, pain control, and patient satisfaction across various surgeries. Below, we summarize key findings and outcomes of ERAS implementation in several major specialties:

3.1 Colorectal, pancreatic and gastric surgery

Colorectal surgery was the cradle of ERAS, and it remains the field with the most robust evidence base for ERAS benefits. Traditional colon resections historically involved lengthy hospitalizations and high morbidity, but ERAS has dramatically changed this scenario. Multiple studies and meta-analyses have confirmed that ERAS significantly reduces postoperative complications and accelerates discharge in colorectal patients [14, 15]. According to the ERAS Society, adopting ERAS pathways in colorectal surgery can reduce postoperative morbidity by approximately 48% compared to conventional care, alongside a median reduction in hospital length of stay of about 2.5 days [14, 15]. These improvements come without compromising safety; in fact, fewer complications (such as infections or thromboembolism) and earlier return of bowel function are typically observed. A comprehensive meta-analysis of 74 randomized trials across various surgeries (many of which were colorectal cases) found that ERAS protocols are associated with significantly shorter hospital stays and fewer overall complications than standard perioperative care [16]. Patients on ERAS pathways after colorectal resections also tend to have earlier mobilization and quicker recovery of normal activities, contributing to higher satisfaction. It is noteworthy that the benefits of ERAS accrue from the entire protocol rather than any single element, underscoring the importance of full pathway compliance in colorectal cases [14, 15]. Over two decades, ERAS has become standard for elective colorectal surgery, showing better outcomes and good tolerance even in elderly or high-risk patients with proper adjustments.

In gastric cancer surgery, especially laparoscopic gastrectomy, ERAS has been shown in meta-analyses to enhance recovery, lower complications, and shorten hospital stay without compromising safety [17, 18]. Though evidence is limited, one study found ERAS in pancreatic cancer surgery reduced complications, hospital stay, and readmissions [19].

3.2 Orthopedic surgery

Enhanced recovery principles are increasingly used in orthopedic surgery, especially total joint arthroplasty, where faster recovery is critical. ERAS improves pain control, early mobilization, and reduces blood loss. A 2023 meta-analysis of 47 studies with ~77,000 patients confirms its benefits [10]. This analysis found that ERAS protocols significantly shortened the length of stay by an average of 2.65 days for joint replacement patients compared to conventional care [10]. Importantly, these faster discharges were achieved without any increase in readmissions or postoperative complications [10]. In fact, ERAS patients had lower rates of blood transfusion (OR ~ 0.40) due to measures like tranexamic acid and careful hemostasis, and even a reduced 30-day mortality by roughly 54% (OR 0.46) relative to controls [10]. Patients in ERAS pathways also reported better pain scores (lower visual analog scale ratings) and improved early range of motion in the new joint, indicating more effective rehabilitation [10]. ERAS enables more patients to return home sooner and regain function faster. In orthopedic surgery, success is linked to regional anesthesia, early mobilization, and nausea control. Widely adopted in joint replacements, meta-analyses show ERAS shortens stays, improves pain control, and increases satisfaction without raising complications [7, 20]. It also eases hospital resource use by freeing beds earlier. Many centers now use ERAS or similar fast-track protocols as standard care. In spine surgery, a review found that ERAS components like multimodal analgesia and early mobilization reduce pain, opioid use, and length of stay [21].

3.3 Thoracic surgery

Patients undergoing thoracic procedures (such as lung resections for cancer) have also benefited from ERAS adaptations. Thoracic surgery traditionally carries significant risks of pulmonary complications and prolonged hospital stays due to thoracotomy pain and chest tube management. ERAS programs for thoracic surgery (sometimes called ERATS—enhanced recovery after thoracic surgery or TERAS) incorporate strategies like minimally invasive video-assisted thoracoscopic surgery (VATS), regional analgesia (thoracic epidurals or nerve blocks), and early chest drain removal to speed recovery. A recent systematic review (2024) of ERAS in general thoracic surgery synthesized results from 30 studies (including four meta-analyses) and concluded that ERAS consistently leads to shorter lengths of stay in thoracic patients and likely contributes to reduced postoperative morbidity as well [12]. Most studies in the review showed significant reductions in hospital stay with ERAS, even though the degree of complication reduction varied among reports [12]. For instance, with ERAS, many lobectomy patients can be discharged in 2–3 days if uncomplicated, compared to a nearly week-long stay under older care models. Postoperative pain control is dramatically improved by using multimodal analgesia (epidurals or intercostal blocks combined with non-opioid analgesics), which in turn facilitates coughing, breathing exercises, and ambulation—critical factors in preventing atelectasis and pneumonia. ERAS has also emphasized preoperative patient education in thoracic surgery, teaching incentive spirometry and nutritional preparation, which helps patients recover faster. While the review noted some variability in outcomes, the overall trend was positive, and no studies indicated any harm from ERAS [12]. In practice, centers implementing ERAS in thoracic surgery have reported fewer incidences of prolonged air leaks, earlier return of pulmonary function, and high patient satisfaction owing to better pain control. With the release of formal ERAS guidelines for lung surgery in recent years, the thoracic surgery community is increasingly standardizing these practices, expecting continued improvements in both clinical outcomes and efficiency of care.

3.4 Gynecologic surgery

ERAS has been widely adopted in gynecologic oncology and major benign gynecologic surgeries, yielding significant gains in recovery and hospital metrics. Women undergoing procedures such as colorectal resection for ovarian cancer debulking, hysterectomy (open or minimally invasive), or pelvic surgery benefit from ERAS elements tailored to their needs (e.g., avoiding bowel prep in gynecologic oncology and thromboprophylaxis in cancer patients). A 2021 systematic review and meta-analysis of ERAS in gynecologic oncology (covering 31 studies with over 6700 patients) provides robust evidence for the effectiveness of ERAS in this field [22]. The meta-analysis found that ERAS implementation was associated with a reduction in hospital length of stay by about 1.6 days on average (95% CI: 1.2–2.1 days) for gynecologic cancer surgeries [22]. More importantly, ERAS patients had significantly fewer complications—a 32% reduction in overall postoperative complications (OR 0.68) compared to those on traditional pathways [22]. There was also a notable 20% decrease in 30-day readmission rates in ERAS groups (OR 0.80) [22], dispelling concerns that faster discharges might lead to more readmissions. Crucially, these improvements did not come at the cost of safety: there was no increase in mortality with ERAS (if anything, a non-significant trend toward lower mortality was observed) [22]. ERAS patients report lower pain scores, reduced opioid use, earlier bowel recovery, and greater satisfaction due to faster recovery and active care involvement. A gynecologic oncology meta-analysis also noted economic benefits, with average cost savings of $2129 per patient [22]. Given these benefits, leading cancer centers now routinely use ERAS for surgeries like ovarian cytoreduction and radical hysterectomy. Similar outcomes are seen in benign procedures, such as endometriosis and fibroid surgery, with shorter stays and better pain control. ERAS is now widely endorsed as standard care in gynecologic surgery by groups like the ERAS® Society and ACOG.

3.5 Urologic surgery

Major urologic surgeries like radical cystectomy and prostatectomy traditionally involve long stays and high complication rates. ERAS protocols in urology—featuring early tube removal, epidural analgesia, ambulation, and no bowel prep—have gained traction. A 2023 meta-analysis of 25 studies (~4000 patients) showed ERAS significantly improved outcomes in cystectomy, with shorter hospital stays (SMD −0.79) and earlier bowel recovery (SMD −1.16) [13]. ERAS was linked to fewer overall (OR ~ 0.76) and serious complications, lower transfusion rates, and reduced 30-day readmissions, without affecting mortality or long-term cancer outcomes [13]. Practically, ERAS enables earlier discharge and lowers rates of postoperative ileus. Similar benefits are seen in other urologic surgeries—ERAS for prostatectomy enables next-day discharge with minimal pain, while protocols for partial nephrectomy and nephroureterectomy reduce opioid use and hospital stay. Urologic surgeons have embraced ERAS as a way to safely hasten recovery and reduce complications in procedures that traditionally carried high morbidity [13]. As with other fields, success in urologic ERAS is driven by multidisciplinary coordination—involving urologists, anesthesiologists, nurses, and physiotherapists—to ensure early mobilization, careful fluid/pain management, and close postoperative monitoring. The evidence base, spanning multiple meta-analyses, confirms that ERAS in urology improves patient outcomes and should be considered the new standard pathway for major surgeries like cystectomy [13].

3.6 Other specialties

Beyond the areas above, ERAS principles have been extended to many other surgical domains.

Hepatopancreatobiliary (HPB) surgery (liver and pancreatic resections) is one such field—traditionally high-risk operations with long recoveries—where ERAS has begun to show benefits. For instance, centers using ERAS for liver resection report shorter ICU and ward stays, earlier return of liver function, and reduced complications like liver insufficiency. A systematic review in liver surgery found significantly lower hospital costs and length of stay with ERAS [23].

Vascular surgery (e.g., elective open aortic aneurysm repair) and neurosurgery (e.g., spine surgery, craniotomy) are also exploring ERAS-like pathways or fast-track programs, although evidence is still emerging. Even cardiac surgery programs have incorporated ERAS elements (often termed "fast-track cardiac care"), emphasizing early extubation, mobilization, and multimodal analgesia, resulting in shorter ICU stays [24].

While the evidence for ERAS in pediatric surgery is more limited, a review article suggested that the adoption of ERAS principles, such as preoperative optimization, minimally invasive techniques, and early feeding, may be beneficial in improving postoperative outcomes in children undergoing various surgical procedures [25].

The ERAS Society has published guidelines for perioperative care in cardiac surgery, which include recommendations for anesthetic management, pain control, and early mobilization [26]. A systematic review found that the adoption of ERAS protocols in heart valve surgery can reduce postoperative complications and promote earlier recovery [27].

The general pattern is consistent: when perioperative care is standardized and improved *via* ERAS principles, patients tend to recover sooner and with fewer complications, regardless of the surgical specialty [2]. Of course, each specialty adapts the ERAS guidelines to its unique needs (for example, neurosurgical ERAS might focus on early neurological assessments and avoiding excess fluid that could increase intracranial pressure). While ERAS may not be equally easy to implement in every field (some surgeries have constraints that delay certain ERAS elements), the trend of multidisciplinary, protocol-driven care improving outcomes holds true widely.

In summary, across surgical disciplines, ERAS protocols have demonstrated faster convalescence, reduced morbidity, and improved patient experience. Patients benefit from fewer days in the hospital and a quicker return to normal life, with no increase in readmission or mortality rates in ERAS programs [22]. In many cases, ERAS has actually reduced mortality and serious complications by optimizing every step of care [10]. Patients also report higher satisfaction and quality of life, as their pain is better controlled and they are more actively involved in their recovery [1, 8]. These consistent positive outcomes across specialties underscore that the fundamental concept of ERAS—minimizing the physical and psychological stress of surgery through coordinated, evidence-based care—is broadly applicable and effective. The next section will examine how these clinical improvements translate into operational and economic benefits for hospitals, and why ERAS is as much a quality improvement initiative as it is a clinical protocol.

4. Effects on patient recovery across surgical specialties

Adopting ERAS protocols improves both patient outcomes and hospital efficiency. By accelerating recovery and lowering complications, ERAS positively affects key operational metrics, length of stay, bed turnover, resource use, and cost. In short, what benefits patient recovery is that it also enhances hospital performance. The following section explores ERAS's impact on healthcare efficiency and quality from a systems perspective.

4.1 Reduced length of stay (LOS) and bed turnover

One of the most immediate effects of ERAS is a shorter postoperative hospital stay for patients, as evidenced by numerous studies across specialties. When patients go home sooner, hospitals free up beds more quickly for new admissions, effectively increasing bed turnover and capacity. This is critical in high-demand surgical units where waiting times for surgery can be long. ERAS has been explicitly credited with improving bed turnover efficiency in surgical wards [4]. For example, if an average colorectal surgery patient's stay drops from ~7 to ~4 days under ERAS, over the course of a year, a surgical unit can treat significantly more patients with the same bed infrastructure. Faster bed turnover also means fewer elective surgeries are delayed due to a lack of inpatient beds. However, it is important that reduced LOS is achieved without a spike in readmissions—a balance ERAS has generally maintained by improving overall recovery (as noted, readmission rates often stay the same or even decrease under ERAS care) [22]. In effect, ERAS allows hospitals to increase throughput while maintaining or enhancing the quality of care. This improved efficiency can be especially beneficial in publicly funded health systems or busy centers where bed availability is a limiting factor for surgical scheduling. It also has a positive impact on emergency departments and intensive care units, since fewer complications and shorter ward stays reduce downstream bottlenecks in the hospital.

4.2 Cost reduction and economic benefits

A consistent finding in ERAS research is the reduction of healthcare costs associated with surgical care [1, 2, 8]. Shorter hospital stays directly lower hospitalization costs (fewer inpatient days and less ICU time). Additionally, by preventing complications (which are expensive to manage and often require interventions or prolonged care), ERAS curtails the costs of postoperative morbidity. Several economic analyses and meta-analyses have demonstrated substantial cost savings from ERAS. For instance, in gynecologic oncology surgeries, implementing ERAS saved an average of $2000+ per patient in direct costs, as mentioned earlier [22]. In liver surgery, a meta-analysis showed significantly lower hospital costs in the ERAS group compared to standard care [23]. Similar trends have been reported in colorectal and orthopedic surgeries—one study noted a roughly 30% reduction in total hospital costs for ERAS patients after colorectal resection [23]. The cost savings stem not only from reduced LOS but also from lower rates of interventions like transfusions, less need for expensive ICU stays, and fewer readmissions or reoperations. From a broader perspective, when patients recover faster and healthier, they may require less post-discharge rehabilitation or home care, translating to indirect cost savings for the healthcare system and society. Importantly, these savings do not imply cutting corners; rather, they result from delivering better care upfront. By investing in prophylactic and streamlined care (e.g., proper analgesia, prophylaxis, early mobilization with physical therapy), hospitals avoid the far higher costs of treating complications or prolonged recoveries. Many hospital administrators thus view ERAS as a high-value proposition—an approach that improves outcomes and reduces cost, aligning with value-based healthcare goals. Indeed, ERAS is often highlighted as a prime example of how quality improvement can drive cost-efficiency in tandem [4].

4.3 Improved healthcare quality metrics

ERAS protocols, by virtue of standardizing best practices, inherently improve compliance with evidence-based care processes. This can positively influence quality metrics that hospitals track, such as surgical site infection rates, venous thromboembolism rates, patient satisfaction scores, and early mobilization rates. For example, a hospital-wide ERAS initiative might track the percentage of patients who ambulate on postoperative day 0 or 1, or who receive appropriate multimodal analgesia, as internal quality indicators. High adherence to these processes correlates with better patient outcomes (fewer pneumonias, fewer pressure ulcers, and better pain control). Many institutions have reported improved patient satisfaction and experience after ERAS implementation [28, 29]. Patients often report smoother recoveries, better pain control, and coordinated care, reflected in higher satisfaction scores. ERAS also improves readmission rates and patient-reported quality-of-life outcomes. Early mobilization and feeding lower the risk of complications, including healthcare-associated infections. These improvements enhance a hospital's care quality profile, and many accreditation bodies now encourage ERAS as a standard for perioperative care.

4.4 Staff and workflow efficiency

Operationally, ERAS enables more predictable and efficient workflows through standardized protocols. Perioperative teams—surgeons, anesthesiologists, nurses, physiotherapists, and dietitians—coordinate more effectively, with each member aware of their role and timing. For example, nurses can plan mobilization, therapists schedule early sessions, and pharmacists prepare analgesia regimens in advance. This clarity improves both patient care and staff satisfaction by reducing variability and ad-hoc decisions. As recovery becomes more streamlined, units may see fewer complications, less overcrowding, and smoother transitions from surgery to discharge, aided by defined milestones. From a management view, this results in more reliable surgical services, better resource use, and potentially reduced overtime. While staff may initially worry ERAS adds tasks, in practice, patients recovering well often require less intensive care, lightening the overall workload. These benefits typically emerge fully once the initial implementation phase is complete.

In summary, ERAS enhances hospital efficiency and care quality by shortening stays, increasing bed turnover, reducing costs, and improving patient outcomes. It lowers complication rates and boosts quality of life, resulting in both clinical and economic gains [4, 30, 31]. This alignment of patient-centered care with system efficiency makes ERAS highly attractive to administrators and policy-makers. In value-based healthcare, ERAS stands out as a strategy that delivers better outcomes at equal or lower costs. For hospitals, adopting ERAS also signals a commitment to advanced, high-quality surgical care.

5. Implementing ERAS protocols hospital-wide: Strategies and considerations

While the benefits of ERAS are well-documented, the successful implementation of ERAS protocols across a hospital or health system requires careful planning, multidisciplinary collaboration, and strong leadership. Hospital administrators and perioperative leaders play a crucial role in facilitating this change. Here we outline key strategies and considerations for implementing ERAS on a broad scale:

5.1 Multidisciplinary ERAS team and leadership

A critical first step is to establish a dedicated ERAS committee or working group that includes all relevant stakeholders—surgeons from various specialties, anesthesiologists, nurses, nurse anesthetists, physiotherapists, dietitians, pharmacists, and hospital administrators. This multidisciplinary team will be responsible for developing or adapting ERAS protocols, educating staff, and monitoring outcomes. Successful ERAS programs often identify "ERAS champions" in each department—clinicians who are passionate about the approach and can lead by example and address specialty-specific issues [1]. Leadership support is paramount: hospital executives and department heads should visibly back the ERAS initiative, helping to create a collaborative culture that encourages change [32]. A collaborative leadership culture means that the facility's leadership and the interdisciplinary team work in partnership, breaking down silos that traditionally separate surgery, anesthesia, and nursing. Regular meetings of the ERAS committee help maintain momentum, troubleshoot problems, and ensure everyone is aligned with the goals. Clear leadership also helps in allocating necessary resources (for example, funding for staff training or purchasing warming devices for the OR). As one implementation guide noted, "the first and foremost thing needed is for a surgeon, the hospital, or a specialty to find a multidisciplinary care team that is engaged"—this forms the backbone of ERAS implementation from the start [33]. Engaged teams are better able to develop standardized order sets, streamline communication, and maintain accountability for ERAS elements.

5.2 Education and engagement of staff and patients

Education is a linchpin of ERAS implementation. All healthcare providers involved need to understand the rationale behind each ERAS element and how to execute it. This often involves formal training sessions, workshops, or webinars for surgeons, anesthesiology staff, nursing staff, and physical therapy teams on ERAS principles and protocols. Early in an implementation, hospitals may conduct in-service training on topics like new anesthesia protocols (e.g., how to manage epidurals in an ERAS setting), early mobilization techniques, or nutritional care plans. It is vital to address any misconceptions—for instance, long-held beliefs about fasting or bed rest—by presenting evidence that supports the new practices [1, 5, 8]. Engaging staff by explaining how ERAS will improve patient care (and even make their jobs easier in the long run) helps gain buy-in. In addition to staff, patient education is equally important. ERAS programs usually include preoperative counseling for patients where the care team explains the ERAS pathway: patients learn about the importance of, for example, drinking carbohydrate fluids before surgery, getting up soon after surgery, and participating in their recovery. When patients understand the "why" and "how" of ERAS, they are more likely to cooperate with early mobilization and oral intake, which improves compliance and outcomes. Many hospitals provide patient education materials (booklets or videos) as part of the ERAS pathway [34]. Engagement of patients and families fosters a partnership mentality—patients become active contributors to their recovery rather than passive recipients of care. Overall, continuous education ensures that everyone is on the same page regarding ERAS protocols, which is critical for consistency. As noted in an ERAS implementation guide, successful adoption depends on patient and staff education and engagement, along with leadership support and continuous data feedback [33].

5.3 Pilot programs and phased implementation

Implementing ERAS hospital-wide can be complex, so a phased approach often works best. Many institutions start by piloting ERAS in one surgical specialty or unit (for instance, colorectal surgery or gynecologic surgery) where there is both a high need and a group of enthusiastic supporters. This allows the hospital to work through initial challenges on a smaller scale, develop best practices, and demonstrate success. Early wins from a pilot—such as reduced length of stay or improved patient feedback—can then be used to build momentum and justify expanding ERAS to other specialties. This is aligned with change management principles: start small, learn, and then scale up. For example, a hospital might implement ERAS in colorectal and orthopedic departments in the first year, then add more specialties (like urology and gynecology) the next year. During expansion, protocols are adapted to each specialty's needs while keeping the core ERAS philosophy intact. Hospital management should ensure that lessons learned from one department (e.g., how to effectively track compliance, or how to deal with certain barriers) are shared across departments to avoid reinventing the wheel. Phased implementation also helps in resource allocation—the hospital can focus training and resources on the pilot area first, then gradually invest in others. It is crucial to maintain a sense of standardization across the hospital even as different specialties adapt specifics; having a central ERAS committee overseeing all specialties can maintain coherence of the overall program.

5.4 Integration into hospital systems and pathways

For ERAS to be sustainable, its practices should be embedded into the hospital's standard operating procedures. This can include updating electronic medical record (EMR) systems to incorporate ERAS order sets (for example, a standardized postoperative order set that automatically prompts for multimodal analgesia, diet advancement, DVT prophylaxis, etc., according to ERAS protocol). Utilizing the EMR to remind and track compliance can significantly ease the implementation. Some hospitals develop ERAS dashboards in their EMR that flag if certain elements have not been completed by certain times. Additionally, aligning ERAS with existing hospital initiatives—such as surgical safety checklists or infection prevention programs—can create synergies. For instance, ERAS protocols that emphasize antibiotic prophylaxis and normothermia align with surgical infection reduction protocols. Another practical step is to incorporate ERAS elements into pre-admission testing clinics or preoperative surgical home models so that optimization (smoking cessation programs, nutrition shakes, etc.) is handled systematically. Hospitals might also need to adjust scheduling: for example, ensuring physical therapists are available on weekends if patients are mobilizing early, or providing meals at odd hours if patients are allowed to eat soon after surgery. From a management view, these adjustments require coordination between departments like dietary services, physiotherapy, and nursing administration.

5.5 Monitoring, data audit, and continuous improvement

A hallmark of ERAS programs is the use of data to drive improvement. Hospitals should establish metrics to monitor the progress and impact of ERAS. Common metrics include average postoperative LOS for each procedure (comparing before vs. after ERAS), complication rates (infection, ileus, etc.), readmission rates, patient satisfaction scores, and compliance rates with each ERAS element (e.g., percentage of patients who received carbohydrate loading or percentage who ambulated on day 1). Regular auditing of these metrics helps identify areas where the protocol is not being followed or is not working as expected. Many ERAS programs use audit results to provide feedback to clinical teams—for example, if one element like "early removal of urinary catheter" has low compliance, the team can investigate why (perhaps unclear orders or fear of urinary retention) and address it. Hospitals may also participate in external ERAS registries or benchmarking programs to compare their outcomes with peers and learn best practices. Continuous quality improvement cycles (Plan-Do-Study-Act cycles) are often employed: implement changes, measure outcomes, refine the protocol, and repeat. This iterative process ensures that the ERAS program does not stagnate and continues to optimize care. The use of data also helps maintain staff motivation; showing clinicians concrete improvements (such as a graph of reduced LOS or complications since ERAS began) reinforces the value of their efforts and encourages continued adherence. In sum, a data-driven approach and willingness to refine protocols are key to sustained ERAS success—as one meta-analysis noted, future efforts should focus on improving implementation and compliance with ERAS guidelines to further improve patient outcomes [16].

5.6 Patient-centered adjustments

Hospital-wide implementation must also recognize that ERAS is not a one-size-fits-all formula; flexibility and individualization are sometimes necessary. Administrative protocols should empower clinicians to tailor ERAS elements when needed (while still adhering to the spirit of ERAS). For example, an elderly frail patient might need a modified mobilization plan or an extra day in hospital, or a patient with specific cultural dietary needs might require alternative nutritional planning. Having a mechanism for case-by-case evaluation—such as an ERAS coordinator or advanced practice nurse who can adjust protocols safely—can ensure that ERAS benefits are extended to as many patients as appropriate without being overly rigid. The key is maintaining the balance between standardization and personalization. Hospitals can incorporate patient feedback into ERAS refinements; for instance, if patients consistently report a particular issue (like anxiety about early discharge), the program can respond by enhancing education or support for that aspect. Ultimately, implementing ERAS hospital-wide is about creating a patient-centered culture of recovery, where every team member is oriented toward the goal of safely getting the patient back to normal life as quickly as possible.

In conclusion, implementing ERAS protocols requires a structured change management approach: build a committed multidisciplinary team, educate and engage all stakeholders, integrate protocols into daily practice, and continually monitor and improve. As one article described, ERAS implementation is a process that evolves from "creation of an engaging story, leadership, a climate supportive of the change, a trial in one specialty, and sustained change with continued improvement," and it faces challenges such as traditional mindsets and staff concerns that must be addressed with communication and data [1, 8, 28, 33]. Hospitals that navigate this process successfully can achieve the full promise of ERAS—better outcomes for patients and more efficient care delivery.

6. Challenges and barriers in ERAS adoption

Despite the clear advantages of ERAS, healthcare organizations often encounter a variety of challenges and barriers when implementing these protocols. Understanding and addressing these barriers is crucial for ERAS programs to reach their full potential. The obstacles can be cultural, logistical, and clinical in nature:

6.1 Cultural resistance and mindset

One of the primary challenges is changing long-standing habits and beliefs among healthcare providers. Surgery and perioperative care have traditions that some staff are reluctant to alter. For example, some surgeons or nurses may initially resist practices like not using a nasogastric tube or allowing feeding on the first postoperative day, because it contradicts what they were trained to do for decades. As the American Association of Nurse Anesthesiology ERAS implementation guide noted, "despite the proven successes of ERAS, implementation challenges exist due to long-held team member and patient opinions of how things should be done. There are some who believe that traditional care works just fine" [8]. These beliefs include outdated views on prolonged fasting, strict bed rest, or heavy reliance on opioids for pain—practices that ERAS challenges with evidence. Overcoming this resistance requires persistent education and showcasing data from literature and one's own institution to convince skeptics that the new ways are indeed better. Additionally, some staff may feel that new protocols are a critique of their past care ("were we doing it wrong all these years?"). Leadership and ERAS champions need to navigate these conversations with respect and focus on the shared goal of improving patient care. Celebrating early successes (like a patient recovering notably faster) and highlighting positive feedback can help win over doubters. It often helps to have respected surgeon and nurse champions within each specialty advocate for ERAS; peer influence can be more effective than top-down mandates in shifting culture.

6.2 Staff workload and resource concerns

Another common barrier is the perception that ERAS will increase workload or require resources the hospital does not have. For instance, nurses might worry that encouraging patients to ambulate or eat so soon will demand more of their time, or anesthesiologists might be concerned that doing nerve blocks and epidurals routinely will lengthen turnover times. Staff already "overwhelmed with workload and time constraints may feel that the ERAS program will add additional strain and complexity to their day" [8]. In some cases, additional resources are indeed needed—for example, more physical therapists to assist with mobilization, or stocking new items like carbohydrate drinks and warming blankets. Hospitals must be prepared to invest initially (which can be justified by the downstream cost savings and outcome improvements) and to reassure staff that support will be provided. Often, these concerns can be mitigated by explaining that while some tasks are new, others will diminish (for example, if patients have fewer complications, there will be fewer crises or lengthy wound care needs). Cross-training and teamwork can distribute the workload: for example, involving family members in mobilizing patients or having physical therapy technicians help. Showing staff the efficiency benefits (like patients discharged earlier, meaning fewer high-acuity patients on the floor at a given time) can reframe the narrative—ERAS is not about doing more tasks, but about doing tasks differently for a better end result.

6.3 Knowledge gaps and training needs

Inadequate knowledge of ERAS principles among healthcare providers is a significant barrier, especially in settings where ERAS is new. A Knowledge, Attitudes, and Practices (KAP) study in a resource-limited hospital revealed "limited awareness of ERAS protocols" among perioperative staff—for example, only 45.7% of participants were familiar with updated fasting (Nil Per Os) guidelines, and less than half knew about early feeding practices [1]. This indicates that without proper training, many staff might simply not know what ERAS entails or may only be "unknowingly applying some ERAS elements" sporadically [1]. The same study found that despite low specific knowledge, almost all respondents (97.7%) believed ERAS improved care and over 79% felt it reduced hospital costs [1], suggesting that once educated, they are likely to support it. Thus, targeted education and training sessions are needed to close the knowledge gap. If a hospital fails to provide comprehensive training, ERAS protocols might be inconsistently applied or misunderstood. Simulation sessions, protocol booklets, and shadowing in early adopter units are ways to enhance knowledge. Additionally, continuous education (refreshers, updates as protocols evolve) is necessary to maintain knowledge over time, especially with staff turnover.

6.4 Interdisciplinary communication and collaboration

ERAS, by its nature, demands tight coordination across different departments and professionals. Poor communication or siloed practices can hinder implementation. For instance, if anesthesiologists, surgeons, and nurses do not coordinate, an element like multimodal analgesia might fall through the cracks (surgeon expects anesthesia to do a block; anesthesia expects surgeon to order certain meds; nurse is unaware of mobilization plans, etc.). A Frontiers article on ERAS highlighted that effective communication among all disciplines involved in the patient's journey is crucial for success, and noted that insufficient communication and collaboration remain a barrier to successful ERAS implementation [2]. To address this, structured communication channels are needed: multidisciplinary rounds on postoperative patients, handoff protocols that include ERAS goals, and inclusion of ERAS status in shift change reports. The ERAS committee should also facilitate interdepartmental dialog—for example, having anesthesia and surgery agree on a standardized pain management plan rather than each anesthesiologist doing something different. Electronic health record tools can assist communication (shared order sets, flags for ERAS patients, etc.). Building a culture of trust and teamwork is fundamental; each discipline should value the others' contributions to ERAS (e.g., surgeons valuing nurses' role in mobilization, etc.). When communication is optimized, ERAS protocols run smoothly; when it is poor, patients may get mixed messages or incomplete interventions (e.g., a patient might be kept NPO unnecessarily because one team was not aware oral intake was allowed).

6.5 Logistical and resource limitations

Implementing ERAS may face practical resource constraints. In some hospitals, especially those in low-resource settings, infrastructure issues like limited availability of consumables (carb drinks and epidural kits), lack of dedicated physical therapy staff, or insufficient ICU capacity can pose challenges [1]. For example, early mobilization requires enough personnel or assistive devices to help patients walk safely; if a ward is understaffed, this becomes difficult. Similarly, ensuring patients drink a pre-op carbohydrate drink presupposes the supply chain and processes to give it on time. In such cases, hospitals need to creatively allocate resources or start ERAS in areas where it's most feasible first. The Rwanda ERAS introduction study pointed out issues like infrastructure constraints and limited ICU capacity as barriers, but demonstrated that adaptation to local context (like focusing on elements that cost little, such as early feeding and mobilization) can still yield benefits [1]. Limited data systems can hinder ERAS monitoring, especially in smaller hospitals. External support, collaboration, and phased implementation can help. Many ERAS elements—like education, early ambulation, and tube avoidance—are low-cost, making them feasible even in resource-limited settings.

6.6 Patient factors and expectations

Not all patients readily embrace ERAS without hesitation. Some patients have their own preconceived notions (e.g., older patients might be fearful of getting out of bed too soon, or might equate a longer hospital stay with better care). Managing patient expectations and addressing concerns is necessary to prevent patients themselves from unintentionally hindering ERAS goals. Additionally, certain patient populations—such as the very frail, those with many comorbidities, or those undergoing extremely extensive surgeries—may have heterogeneous outcomes under ERAS and might need protocol modifications [11]. For instance, an ERAS pathway might typically aim for discharge on postoperative day 3, but an elderly patient with limited home support might need an extra day or two; rigid insistence on protocol in such cases could be counterproductive. Therefore, flexibility and clinical judgment remain important. Some studies have noted that high-risk groups benefit from ERAS but perhaps not as dramatically as lower-risk patients, suggesting a need to tailor certain ERAS elements (like more gradual mobilization or extended monitoring) for them [11]. Another patient-related barrier is adherence: after discharge, ERAS encourages ongoing recovery measures (like exercises and nutrition)—if patients do not adhere, they could be readmitted. Providing clear instructions and follow-up (e.g., phone calls or telehealth check-ins post-discharge) can improve patient adherence and allay any post-discharge issues early. In summary, patient-specific factors require an individualized approach within the ERAS framework—something hospitals must incorporate into their protocols and education.

6.7 Compliance and sustaining change

Initiating ERAS is one challenge; sustaining high compliance long-term is another. Over time, there can be protocol drift—as new staff come in or initial enthusiasm wanes, certain ERAS elements might be neglected. Regular auditing and feedback, as mentioned earlier, are key to preventing this. Some meta-analyses (like the gynecologic oncology one) intriguingly found no clear difference in outcomes based on the number of ERAS elements implemented or reported compliance [22, 28], but this should not be taken to mean compliance is unimportant. On the contrary, high compliance is generally correlated with better outcomes in many ERAS studies, but measuring compliance accurately can be difficult. The challenge for management is to keep ERAS as a priority amidst many other hospital initiatives. Turnover of champions or leaders can also threaten continuity. Thus, embedding ERAS into institutional policy (for example, making certain ERAS order sets the default for relevant surgeries, or including ERAS metrics in departmental performance reviews) can help maintain focus. It is also effective to periodically update and refresh the program—incorporating new evidence or expanding ERAS to new procedures—which keeps the team engaged and the program dynamic.

In tackling these challenges, transparency and communication are vital. Hospitals have found that actively addressing concerns and barriers through data and open communication is critical prior to implementing the ERAS program [8, 33]. For example, if nurses worry about workload, show them data from elsewhere that nurse workload did not increase, or patient outcomes improved, such that overall effort was less frantic. If surgeons doubt a specific element, pilot it and share the positive patient feedback or outcome improvement. Some barriers, like limited awareness, are relatively straightforward to fix *via* education; others, like ingrained culture, take persistent effort and sometimes generational change. The presence of external guidelines and endorsements (e.g., ERAS Society guidelines and or national surgical society recommendations) can bolster the case, giving local implementers the authoritative backing to counter resistance.

Finally, it is worth recognizing that not every barrier can be eliminated; rather, they can be managed. ERAS implementation is a journey of continuous improvement. Even after initial challenges are overcome, new ones might emerge (for instance, as ERAS extends to new surgical areas or as patient populations change). Hospitals must remain adaptive. The encouraging reality, shown in many case studies, is that once a critical mass of success is achieved—when staff see patients doing better and hospital metrics improving—the ERAS approach tends to become self-sustaining. What was once viewed skeptically as a radical change becomes the "new normal" of care. At that point, the culture shifts from "why do we need ERAS?" to "why wouldn't we always do it this way?"—which is the ultimate overcoming of the initial barriers.

7. Conclusion

Enhanced recovery after surgery (ERAS) protocols have emerged as a transformative force in surgical care, marrying the objectives of improved patient recovery with enhanced hospital efficiency. Through a multimodal, multidisciplinary approach, ERAS effectively reduces the physiologic stress of surgery, which translates into tangible benefits: patients experience fewer complications, better pain control, shorter hospital stays, and faster returns to normal function, all while maintaining or even improving satisfaction with their care. Across numerous surgical specialties—from colorectal and orthopedic surgery to thoracic, gynecologic, and urologic procedures—ERAS has consistently demonstrated superior outcomes compared to traditional perioperative management [22]. These clinical gains have been paralleled by organizational advantages such as lower healthcare costs and more efficient use of hospital beds and staff resources [23]. In an era where healthcare systems strive for high-quality, cost-effective care, ERAS stands out as a paradigm that achieves both aims.

From the hospital management perspective, implementing ERAS is both a challenge and an opportunity. It requires upfront investment in planning, education, and culture change, but the payoff is significant in terms of quality improvement and operational performance. The key to success is fostering an institutional culture of collaboration and continuous improvement—surgeons, anesthesiologists, nurses, and allied health professionals working in concert toward common ERAS goals, supported by leadership and guided by data. Hospitals that have embraced ERAS report that it catalyzes broader improvements: it encourages the adoption of evidence-based practices, improves interdisciplinary communication, and focuses attention on the entire perioperative patient journey rather than isolated silos of care [2]. In many ways, ERAS can serve as a model for other quality initiatives, illustrating how systematic, patient-centered changes can elevate outcomes.

Looking forward, the ongoing evolution of ERAS will likely involve refinement and expansion. As research continues, new evidence will further optimize individual ERAS elements (e.g., novel analgesic techniques or enhanced prehabilitation strategies) and extend ERAS principles to specialties not yet fully covered (such as emergency surgeries or transplant surgery). The concept of precision ERAS is emerging, recognizing that protocols may be tailored to specific patient subgroups for maximal

DOI: http://dx.doi.org/10.5772/intechopen.1011649

benefit [11]. Additionally, the focus is shifting toward improving implementation science—ensuring that the known benefits of ERAS are realized broadly in practice. This includes addressing disparities (so that ERAS is not limited to high-resource centers alone) and improving patient engagement and follow-up after discharge. The meta-analysis by Sauro et al. emphasized that future efforts should concentrate on improving implementation and compliance to unlock the full potential of ERAS in improving patient outcomes [16]. Hospital administrators and clinicians will need to remain vigilant in sustaining the ERAS gains, continually educating new staff, and adapting to feedback and new insights.

In conclusion, the impact of ERAS protocols on healthcare quality is profound: they represent a win-win scenario in which patients recover better and faster, and hospitals utilize their resources more effectively. The journey of ERAS from a bold idea in colorectal surgery to a global standard of perioperative care in multiple disciplines is a testament to the power of evidence-based, coordinated care. By prioritizing both the human aspects (patient well-being, staff engagement) and the system aspects (efficiency, cost-effectiveness), ERAS exemplifies holistic healthcare improvement. For any institution aiming to enhance its surgical services, ERAS offers a clear roadmap—one that improves the metrics that matter most, from complication rates to patient smiles to balance sheets. As the surgical community continues to refine ERAS and overcome implementation challenges, we can expect further advancements in how we care for surgical patients, ultimately leading to a new baseline of excellence in perioperative care and hospital management in the years to come.

Author details

Ömer Faruk Sağlam
Thoracic Surgery, Tokat State Hospital, Tokat, Turkey

*Address all correspondence to: mrfrksglm@gmail.com

References

[1] Nyundo M, Gasakure M, Muhawenayo E, Kayondo K, Banguti P, Twagirumukiza JD, et al. Introducing enhanced recovery after surgery (ERAS) program in Rwanda: A step-by-step approach from KAP study to protocol development and preliminary implementation. BMC Surgery. 2025;**25**:173. DOI: 10.1186/s12893-025-02909-6

[2] Xu J-j, Tang X-t, Mao M, Yang Q-n, Jiang L-p, Fu W-c, et al. Hospital-mediated realization of enhanced recovery after surgery. Frontiers in Surgery. 2025;**19**(12):1554301. DOI: 10.3389/fsurg.2025.1554301

[3] Wang LH, Zhu RF, Gao C, Wang SL, Shen LZ. Application of enhanced recovery after gastric cancer surgery: An updated meta-analysis. World Journal of Gastroenterology. 2018;**24**:1562-1578. DOI: 10.3748/wjg.v24.i14.1562

[4] Vinklerová K, Zajak J, Čečka F, Páral J, Sedláčková J. Standardized ERAS protocol in liver and pancreatic surgery. Rozhledy v Chirurgii. 2024;**103**:351-357. English. DOI: 10.48095/ccrvch2024351

[5] Gustafsson UO, Scott MJ, Hubner M, Nygren J, Demartines N, Francis N, et al. Guidelines for perioperative care in elective colorectal surgery: Enhanced recovery after surgery (ERAS ®) society recommendations: 2018. World Journal of Surgery. 2019;**43**:659-695. DOI: 10.1007/s00268-018-4844-y

[6] Pearsall EA, McLeod RS. Enhanced recovery after surgery. Surgical Clinics of North America. 2018;**98**:1201-1210. DOI: 10.1016/j.suc.2018.07.007

[7] Ljungqvist O, Scott M, Fearon KC. Enhanced recovery after surgery. JAMA Surgery. 2017;**152**:292-298. DOI: 10.1001/jamasurg.2016.4952

[8] Reede L, Lukyanova V, Chappell D. Enhanced recovery after surgery: Implementation strategies. American Association of Nurse Anesthesiology News Bulletin. 2017;**11**:30-33

[9] Mithany RH, Daniel N, Shahid MH, Aslam S, Abdelmaseeh M, Gerges F, et al. Revolutionizing surgical care: The power of enhanced recovery after surgery (ERAS). Cureus. 2023;**15**:e48795. DOI: 10.7759/cureus.48795

[10] Zhang Q, Chen Y, Li Y, Liu R, Rai S, Li J, et al. Enhanced recovery after surgery in patients after hip and knee arthroplasty: A systematic review and meta-analysis. Postgraduate Medical Journal. 2024;**100**:159-173. DOI: 10.1093/postmj/qgad125

[11] Hirani R, Podder D, Stala O, Mohebpour R, Tiwari RK, Etienne M. Strategies to reduce hospital length of stay: Evidence and challenges. Medicina (Kaunas, Lithuania). 2025;**61**:922. DOI: 10.3390/medicina61050922

[12] Goldblatt JG, Bibo L, Crawford L. Does enhanced recovery after surgery protocols reduce complications and length of stay after thoracic surgery: A systematic review of the literature. Cureus. 2024;**16**:e59918. DOI: 10.7759/cureus.59918

[13] Zhou Y, Li R, Liu Z, Qi W, Lv G, Zhong M, et al. The effect of the enhanced recovery after surgery program on radical cystectomy: A meta-analysis and systematic review. Frontiers in Surgery. 2023;**10**:1101098. DOI: 10.3389/fsurg.2023.1101098

[14] Spanjersberg WR, Reurings J, Keus F, van Laarhoven CJ. Fast track surgery versus conventional recovery strategies for colorectal surgery. Cochrane Database of Systematic Reviews. 2011;**2**:CD007635. DOI: 10.1002/14651858.CD007635.pub2

[15] Varadhan KK, Lobo DN. A meta-analysis of randomised controlled trials of intravenous fluid therapy in major elective open abdominal surgery: Getting the balance right. The Proceedings of the Nutrition Society. 2010;**69**:488-498. DOI: 10.1017/S0029665110001734

[16] Sauro KM, Smith C, Ibadin S, Thomas A, Ganshorn H, Bakunda L, et al. Enhanced recovery after surgery guidelines and hospital length of stay, readmission, complications, and mortality: A meta-analysis of randomized clinical trials. JAMA Network Open. 2024;**7**:e2417310. DOI: 10.1001/jamanetworkopen.2024.17310

[17] Li MZ, Wu WH, Li L, Zhou XF, Zhu HL, Li JF, et al. Is ERAS effective and safe in laparoscopic gastrectomy for gastric carcinoma? A meta-analysis. World Journal of Surgical Oncology. 2018;**16**:17. DOI: 10.1186/s12957-018-1309-6

[18] Li Z, Wang Q, Li B, Bai B, Zhao Q. Influence of enhanced recovery after surgery programs on laparoscopy-assisted gastrectomy for gastric cancer: A systematic review and meta-analysis of randomized control trials. World Journal of Surgical Oncology. 2017;**15**:207. DOI: 10.1186/s12957-017-1271-8

[19] Agarwal V, Divatia JV. Enhanced recovery after surgery in liver resection: Current concepts and controversies. Korean Journal of Anesthesiology. 2019;**72**:119-129. DOI: 10.4097/kja.d.19.00010

[20] Ljungqvist O, Hubner M. Enhanced recovery after surgery-ERAS-principles, practice and feasibility in the elderly. Aging Clinical and Experimental Research. 2018;**30**:249-252. DOI: 10.1007/s40520-018-0905-1

[21] Dietz N, Sharma M, Adams S, Alhourani A, Ugiliweneza B, Wang D, et al. Enhanced recovery after surgery (ERAS) for spine surgery: A systematic review. World Neurosurgery. 2019;**130**:415-426. DOI: 10.1016/j.wneu.2019.06.181

[22] Bisch SP, Jago CA, Kalogera E, Ganshorn H, Meyer LA, Ramirez PT, et al. Outcomes of enhanced recovery after surgery (ERAS) in gynecologic oncology—A systematic review and meta-analysis. Gynecologic Oncology. 2021;**161**:46-55. DOI: 10.1016/j.ygyno.2020.12.035

[23] Noba L, Rodgers S, Chandler C, Balfour A, Hariharan D, Yip VS. Enhanced recovery after surgery (ERAS) reduces hospital costs and improve clinical outcomes in liver surgery: A systematic review and meta-analysis. Journal of Gastrointestinal Surgery. 2020;**24**:918-932. DOI: 10.1007/s11605-019-04499-0

[24] Aykut A, Salman N, Demir ZA, Özgök A, Günaydın S. Comparison of propofol and sevoflurane anaesthesia in terms of postoperative nausea-vomiting complication in cardiac surgery patients undergoing enhanced recovery after surgery protocol: A prospective randomized study. Turkish Journal of Anaesthesiology and Reanimation. 2024;**52**:113-121. DOI: 10.4274/TJAR.2024.241622

[25] Roberts K, Brindle M, McLuckie D. Enhanced recovery after surgery in paediatrics: A review of the literature.

BJA Education. 2020;**20**:235-241. DOI: 10.1016/j.bjae.2020.03.004

[26] Engelman DT, Ben Ali W, Williams JB, Perrault LP, Reddy VS, Arora RC, et al. Guidelines for perioperative care in cardiac surgery: Enhanced recovery after surgery society recommendations. JAMA Surgery. 2019;**154**:755-766. DOI: 10.1001/jamasurg.2019.1153

[27] Malvindi PG, Bifulco O, Berretta P, Galeazzi M, Alfonsi J, Cefarelli M, et al. The enhanced recovery after surgery approach in heart valve surgery: A systematic review of clinical studies. Journal of Clinical Medicine. 2024;**13**:2903. DOI: 10.3390/jcm13102903

[28] Marchand GJ, Coriell C, Taher A, King A, Ruther S, Brazil G, et al. Systematic review of the effect of implementing enhanced recovery after surgery on selected attributes of surgical recovery in gynecology. Turkish Journal of Obstetrics and Gynecology. 2021;**18**:245-257. DOI: 10.4274/tjod.galenos.2021.47717

[29] Li D, Jensen CC. Patient satisfaction and quality of life with enhanced recovery protocols. Clinics in Colon and Rectal Surgery. 2019;**32**:138-144. DOI: 10.1055/s-0038-1676480

[30] Moosburner S, Dahlke PM, Neudecker J, Hillebrandt KH, Koch PF, Knitter S, et al. From morbidity reduction to cost-effectiveness: Enhanced recovery after surgery (ERAS) society recommendations in minimal invasive liver surgery. Langenbeck's Archives of Surgery. 2024;**409**:137. DOI: 10.1007/s00423-024-03329-5

[31] Lau CS, Chamberlain RS. Enhanced recovery after surgery programs improve patient outcomes and recovery: A meta-analysis. World Journal of Surgery. 2017;**41**:899-913. DOI: 10.1007/s00268-016-3807-4

[32] Shida D, Tagawa K, Inada K, Nasu K, Seyama Y, Maeshiro T, et al. Modified enhanced recovery after surgery (ERAS) protocols for patients with obstructive colorectal cancer. BMC Surgery. 2017;**17**:18. DOI: 10.1186/s12893-017-0213-2

[33] Fox M. ERAS protocols are proven effective, but implementation is challenging. American College of Surgeons Bulletin. 2025;**110**(5):16-23

[34] Bertocchi E, Barugola G, Masini G, Guerriero M, Menestrina N, Gentile I, et al. iColon, a patient-focused mobile application for perioperative care in colorectal surgery: Results from 444 patients. Journal of Telemedicine and Telecare. 2025;**31**:585-591. DOI: 10.1177/1357633X231203064

Chapter 5

Hospital Management in Iran: Challenges, Opportunities, and the Shift toward Smart Hospitals and AI

Pir Hossein Kolivand

Abstract

Hospital management in Iran faces persistent challenges, including financial constraints, workforce shortages, centralized decision-making, and inefficient resource allocation. In recent years, the emergence of digital health technologies—such as artificial intelligence (AI), the Internet of Things (IoT), and hospital information systems (HIS)—has created new opportunities for the transition toward smart hospitals. This chapter examines the current structure and governance of Iranian hospitals, analyzes the impact of digital transformation and AI integration on operational efficiency and patient care, and explores the benefits and barriers associated with the smart hospital implementation. Findings indicate that AI-driven management and digital platforms can significantly improve diagnostic accuracy, reduce costs, and optimize resource use. However, realizing these benefits requires comprehensive reforms, including decentralization, professionalization of hospital leadership, investment in workforce development, and enhanced integration between public and private sectors. The chapter concludes with practical recommendations for fostering innovation and sustainable development in Iran's hospital system through the adoption of smart hospital strategies.

Keywords: hospital management, smart hospital, artificial intelligence, digital health, Iran

1. Introduction

While hospital managers often do not engage directly with patients, the choices and responsibilities entrusted to them can significantly influence the standard of care delivered to patients. Hospital managers play a particularly pivotal role in the administration of healthcare institutions, for example, in the development of organizational strategy and the implementation of changes and transformations. Through their involvement in these tasks, hospital managers can indirectly shape how care is provided to patients. Their behind-the-scenes role involves guiding organizational policies, managing change, and considering the impact of external factors with the aim of enhancing the quality of care and treatment services [1].

By prioritizing patient needs and addressing any unique requests they may have, hospital managers are capable of delivering patient-centered digital health solutions tailored to patients and their specific requirements. Patients, as individuals with distinct personal needs, should be actively involved in the decision-making process regarding their care. For hospital managers to effectively employ a patient-centered approach, they must show utmost respect for patients and consider both cultural norms and the personal preferences of each patient [2].

Hospital managers play a crucial role in the coordination and organization of patient care services. Many individuals experience a loss of control and vulnerability when they become ill. Coordinating all aspects of care, including aligning clinical care with supportive programs and ancillary services, can help reduce the patients' feelings of vulnerability and helplessness [3].

When healthcare organizations integrate all components of the patient treatment process—from medical services to counseling—the sense of helplessness and frailty that accompanies illness is mitigated. It is therefore essential for hospital managers to oversee collaboration between clinical care and supportive services to ensure patients receive comprehensive support. Consequently, hospital managers must assume a key role in coordinating and leading care providers. They must ensure that digital technologies available within a given healthcare organization are optimally utilized to support patient health and well-being. This coordinating role is especially critical when determining public health programs. When hospital managers supervise the integration of technological tools with clinical care and prioritize patient care, patients benefit both individually and collectively. Well-coordinated and managed healthcare systems that prioritize patient outcomes—particularly in meeting public health needs—are vital and indispensable [4].

Hospital management is a specialized field that encompasses the planning, organization, direction, and control of all aspects of hospital operations to ensure the effective and efficient provision of healthcare services. Often referred to as hospital administration or healthcare management, this discipline is fundamental to the smooth functioning of hospitals and broader health systems. At its core, hospital management involves establishing strong leadership and governance structures, where administrators and department heads set strategic direction, cultivate a positive organizational culture, and oversee the delivery of high-quality patient care [5].

Resource management is another critical component, requiring managers to allocate human, financial, and material resources judiciously to maximize operational efficiency and patient outcomes. This includes overseeing staff recruitment and training, managing budgets, and ensuring the availability of necessary equipment and medicines. Additionally, hospital management is responsible for coordinating a wide range of services—from patient registration and appointment scheduling to clinical care and laboratory operations—ensuring that all departments work cohesively toward shared objectives [6].

A major focus of hospital management is the implementation of systems and policies that promote patient safety and enhance the quality of care, while ensuring compliance with healthcare regulations. Continuous performance improvement is also a hallmark of effective management, involving regular monitoring and evaluation to drive better organizational performance, improve patient satisfaction, and achieve the superior clinical outcomes. Research underscores the importance of strong management practices, linking them to improved patient outcomes, higher satisfaction rates, and reduced mortality. Ultimately, hospital management plays a pivotal role in aligning hospital operations with the institution's mission and goals, fostering innovation, and ensuring the overall success of healthcare organizations [7].

The study then explores the growing impact of artificial intelligence (AI) and digital technologies on hospital performance in Iran. Recent advancements in health technology showcased prominently at events like Iran Health 2025, demonstrating the country's commitment to integrating innovative solutions into healthcare delivery [7].

AI applications are increasingly used for optimizing hospital operations, enhancing diagnostic accuracy, managing patient data, and improving financial and resource management. Private hospitals, in particular, have been early adopters of AI-driven tools, which contribute to improved efficiency and patient outcomes [8].

Moreover, digital transformation efforts aim to establish the interconnected health information systems that facilitate better coordination across healthcare providers. These technological advances align with Iran's broader health system vision for 2025, which emphasizes accountability, innovation, and equity in healthcare services. However, challenges such as limited infrastructure in public hospitals and the need for workforce training remain barriers to widespread AI adoption [9].

2. Structure of hospital management in Iran

Hospital management in Iran is characterized by a complex interplay of public and private sector dynamics, shaped by the country's healthcare infrastructure and ongoing reform efforts. The majority of hospitals are publicly owned and managed by the Ministry of Health and Medical Education, which often results in centralized decision-making and challenges related to resource allocation and operational efficiency. Private hospitals, although fewer, are increasingly adopting advanced management techniques, including artificial intelligence, to enhance financial and operational performance. Leadership and governance in Iranian hospitals face issues such as fragmented authority, limited autonomy, and politicization, which hinder strategic planning and effective management [10].

Resource constraints, including financial limitations, staff shortages, and infrastructural gaps, further complicate hospital operations. While progress has been made in areas like primary healthcare delivery, systematic quality assurance and performance evaluation remain inconsistent. Various reform initiatives, such as decentralization efforts and the introduction of autonomous hospital models, have been implemented with mixed success, often due to inadequate policy support and execution. The professionalization of hospital management through the employment of trained health services managers has contributed positively to organizational culture and patient satisfaction [11].

Despite these advances, challenges persist, including bureaucratic rigidity, fragmented health system coordination, financial instability, and leadership deficits. Innovations such as the integration of AI in private hospitals signal a promising direction for the future, with expectations that these technologies will gradually extend to public institutions. Overall, hospital management in Iran is in a transitional phase, balancing traditional centralized structures with emerging reforms and technological advancements. Yet, it requires comprehensive, evidence-based policy measures to overcome systemic barriers and improve healthcare delivery sustainably [12].

Despite this structure, hospitals in Iran face multiple challenges, including staff shortages, inefficient resource management, and currency fluctuations affecting medical equipment costs.

3. Challenges in hospital management in Iran

Hospital management in Iran faces several critical challenges that impact its overall efficiency and effectiveness. A major issue is the highly centralized and bureaucratic nature of the public hospital system, where decision-making power is concentrated at higher administrative levels, limiting the autonomy of hospital managers. This centralization often results in delays and inefficiencies, as hospitals struggle to respond quickly to local needs and changing circumstances [13].

Leadership and governance also present significant difficulties, with many hospital managers lacking formal training in healthcare administration and facing frequent political interference. Such instability leads to inconsistent strategic planning and weakens accountability within hospital operations. Financial constraints further complicate management efforts, as public hospitals operate with limited budgets, inefficient financial systems, and pressure to reduce costs, which can negatively affect infrastructure development, technology adoption, and staff welfare [14].

Human resource challenges are also prominent, including shortages of skilled personnel, low motivation, unclear job roles, and limited opportunities for professional growth, all of which contribute to staff dissatisfaction and reduced performance. Additionally, the fragmentation of Iran's healthcare system—with poor coordination between public and private sectors and a lack of integrated information systems—creates barriers to effective resource allocation and service delivery [15].

Overcoming these challenges requires comprehensive reforms aimed at decentralizing authority, professionalizing hospital leadership, improving financial management, enhancing workforce training and motivation, and fostering better integration across the health system. Such measures are essential to strengthen hospital management and improve the quality and accessibility of healthcare services in Iran [16]. To address these issues, AI-driven solutions and smart hospital strategies can be highly effective.

4. Smart hospitals

Smart hospitals represent a significant advancement in healthcare delivery by integrating cutting-edge digital technologies to improve operational efficiency, enhance patient care, and optimize hospital management. These facilities leverage a range of tools such as artificial intelligence (AI), the Internet of Things (IoT), electronic health records (EHRs), robotics, telemedicine, and predictive analytics to create interconnected systems that streamline clinical workflows and improve health outcomes [17].

For instance, the Mayo Clinic in Rochester is undergoing a $5 billion campus redevelopment, aiming to blend inpatient, outpatient, and virtual care within a fully digitized environment. This project includes innovative features such as flexible clinical spaces and a logistics center designed to support long-term growth and efficient supply management, reflecting a shift toward "care neighborhoods" that group patients by similar needs to enhance care continuity and coordination [18].

Similarly, Cleveland Clinic employs AI and machine learning to analyze patient data, enabling early and accurate detection of diseases such as cancer. Humber River Hospital in Canada exemplifies a "greenfield" smart hospital, built from the ground up with digital-first infrastructure, including a patient command center for real-time monitoring and management [19].

In contrast, Johns Hopkins represents a "brownfield" hospital that continuously upgrades its existing infrastructure with smart technologies to improve care coordination and efficiency. These examples demonstrate the diversity of smart hospital models, from newly constructed digital campuses to existing institutions progressively adopting intelligent technologies to transform healthcare delivery [20].

4.1 The role of artificial intelligence in smart hospital management

Artificial intelligence is central to the functionality and management of smart hospitals, automating and enhancing a broad spectrum of clinical and administrative tasks. AI algorithms process vast amounts of medical data to support diagnostics, predict patient outcomes, and tailor treatment plans with greater speed and accuracy than traditional methods. Smart hospitals provide numerous benefits, including the following:

- *Enhanced patient information management through Electronic Health Records (EHRs)*: EHRs facilitate comprehensive and accessible patient data, improving care continuity and reducing medical errors. For instance, a 2024 study demonstrated that hospitals integrating EHRs with AI platforms significantly improved diagnostic accuracy and treatment coordination [21].

- *Improved diagnostic accuracy and treatment planning with deep learning algorithms for medical imaging*: AI-driven imaging tools detect subtle abnormalities earlier than human interpretation alone, enabling timely interventions. Research shows that deep learning models applied to radiology reduce diagnostic errors and improve cancer detection rates [22].

- *Reduced hospital costs through optimized drug consumption and shorter patient hospitalization*: Smart hospitals use AI to monitor drug usage patterns and patient responses, minimizing waste and adverse effects. Studies report that these optimizations lead to decreased length of stay and overall cost savings [23].

- *Automation of administrative processes with AI-powered chatbots for appointment scheduling and patient registration*: AI chatbots streamline patient interactions, reduce waiting times, and free administrative staff for more complex tasks. Evidence indicates improved patient satisfaction and operational efficiency following chatbot implementation [24].

- *Remote patient monitoring using telemedicine and wearable medical devices:* Telehealth and IoT-enabled wearables allow continuous monitoring of chronic conditions outside hospital settings, reducing unnecessary admissions and enabling proactive care. Clinical trials confirm the improved outcomes and patient engagement through remote monitoring [25].

- *Intelligent resource management for bed allocation, patient flow prediction, and medical staff scheduling*: AI-driven predictive analytics optimize hospital resources, ensuring timely bed availability and efficient staff deployment. Studies have documented reductions in overcrowding and improved patient throughput in hospitals employing these systems [26].

4.2 Benefits and operational transformation through AI in smart hospitals

The integration of AI within smart hospital management not only advances clinical outcomes but also fundamentally transforms hospital operations. AI-driven analytics equip hospital leaders with data-driven insights to optimize staffing, inventory management, and facility maintenance, leading to cost savings and improved service quality [27].

Robotics, another AI-enabled technology, supports surgical precision, automates medication delivery, and assists in patient care activities such as rehabilitation and sanitation, thereby reducing human error and enhancing patient safety. Telemedicine and remote patient monitoring, powered by AI and IoT, extend hospital services beyond physical facilities, enabling continuous care and reducing unnecessary hospital visits [28].

However, the successful implementation of AI in hospital management requires overcoming challenges related to data security, system interoperability, staff training, and ethical considerations. Despite these hurdles, AI remains a cornerstone technology driving the evolution of smart hospitals into adaptive, efficient, and patient-centered institutions. Literature consistently highlights these benefits, reinforcing AI's critical role in shaping the future of hospital management and healthcare delivery worldwide [29].

4.3 Challenges in implementing smart hospitals

Implementing smart hospitals, while promising significant advancements in healthcare, faces a myriad of complex challenges that span technological, organizational, environmental, and societal domains. These challenges often hinder the full realization of smart hospital potential, necessitating careful planning and multifaceted solutions.

- *Lack of a comprehensive and accepted definition*: A fundamental challenge in smart hospital implementation is the absence of a universally accepted and comprehensive definition. This ambiguity leads to varied interpretations and misconceptions, where many developments touted as "smart" merely digitize existing hospital environments without fully embracing the transformative potential of smart technology. This conceptual vagueness can result in fragmented efforts and a lack of clear objectives, making it difficult to measure progress and achieve cohesive integration of smart solutions [30].

- *Technological infrastructure and integration issues*: The deployment of smart hospital technologies, such as 6G, demands extensive infrastructure upgrades, which include robust network capabilities to support ultra-low latency, high data rates, and massive device connectivity. Existing hospital infrastructure may be inadequate, requiring substantial investments in new hardware like advanced routers, servers, and edge computing devices. The complexity of managing vast amounts of data generated by interconnected devices also necessitates sophisticated data processing and storage solutions. Furthermore, ensuring interoperability between diverse systems and devices from various vendors is a significant hurdle, as seamless data exchange is crucial for effective smart hospital operations [31].

- *High costs and financial barriers*: The financial investment required for implementing smart hospital technologies can be prohibitive, especially for smaller or less-resourced healthcare facilities. Beyond initial infrastructure and hardware costs, there are ongoing expenses for maintenance, software licenses, and system upgrades. The need for continuous advancement and rigorous assessment of new technologies adds to the financial burden, making cost-effectiveness a critical consideration for successful deployment [32].

- *Data privacy, cybersecurity risks, and regulatory gaps*: The extensive use of digital health technologies in smart hospitals significantly increases concerns around data privacy and cybersecurity. Hospitals handle sensitive patient information, making them prime targets for cyberattacks. Ensuring the security of vast amounts of data generated by interconnected devices and systems is paramount. While blockchain technology offers potential solutions for data integrity and privacy through decentralized and immutable ledgers, regulatory and legal frameworks often lag behind technological advancements, creating uncertainty and compliance challenges [33].

- *Human resources and organizational resistance*: Implementing smart hospitals requires significant changes in workflow, skills, and organizational culture, often leading to resistance from healthcare professionals. There is a need for continuous training and change management to equip clinicians and patients alike with the necessary skills to utilize new technologies effectively. Furthermore, a lack of awareness and understanding among stakeholders about the benefits of smart healthcare strategies can hinder adoption. Staff may also fear job displacement due to automation, contributing to a reluctance to embrace new systems [34].

- *Inequitable access to technology*: The benefits of digital health and smart hospitals may not be uniformly distributed, leading to inequities in access to advanced healthcare services. Disparities can arise from socioeconomic factors, geographical location, or lack of digital literacy among certain patient populations. Ensuring that smart hospital solutions are accessible and beneficial to all segments of society is a significant ethical and practical challenge [35].

4.4 Challenges in implementing smart hospitals in Iran

Implementing smart hospitals in Iran involves overcoming a range of technological, organizational, financial, and cultural challenges. Recent studies provide detailed insights into these barriers, which must be addressed to realize the potential of smart healthcare in the country.

4.4.1 Technical and infrastructural limitation

A critical challenge in Iran is the incomplete implementation of foundational technologies required for smart hospitals. Full deployment of Electronic Health Records (EHRs), clinical decision support systems, and Internet of Things (IoT) devices remains limited. Many hospitals lack the necessary networking infrastructure and hardware to support real-time data exchange and AI-driven analytics.

For example, a 2023 study highlighted the need for robust IT infrastructure and adoption of international standards to enable interoperability and efficient data flow across hospital systems. Additionally, sanctions have restricted access to some advanced technologies and hardware, further complicating infrastructure development. These technological gaps hinder the integration of AI and machine learning algorithms essential for smart hospital functions such as predictive analytics and automated monitoring [36].

4.4.2 Financial constraints and resource scarcity

Financial barriers are among the most significant obstacles to smart hospital implementation in Iran. The high costs associated with acquiring, deploying, and maintaining advanced digital health technologies pose a challenge, especially for public hospitals operating under budget constraints. Studies report that insufficient funding limits investments in necessary infrastructure upgrades, staff training, and software licenses. Moreover, ongoing economic sanctions exacerbate these financial difficulties by restricting access to international markets and increasing costs. This financial strain often results in delayed or partial adoption of smart hospital components, impeding the realization of their full benefits [36].

4.4.3 Human resource challenges and workforce training

A shortage of skilled healthcare professionals trained in health informatics and digital technologies is a major impediment. Many healthcare workers and hospital managers lack adequate training to effectively utilize smart hospital systems, leading to underuse or misuse of available technologies. Resistance to change and organizational inertia further complicates adoption. For instance, a 2024 study on e-Health implementation in Iranian hospitals identified resistance among physicians and staff due to unfamiliarity with new systems and concerns about increased workload. Continuous education and capacity-building programs are essential to equip healthcare personnel with the skills necessary for operating and managing smart hospital technologies [37].

4.4.4 Organizational and cultural resistance

Cultural and organizational resistance within healthcare institutions poses a significant barrier. Traditional hierarchical structures and established workflows often conflict with the collaborative and flexible nature required for smart hospital operations. Resistance to change is compounded by a lack of awareness about the benefits of smart technologies among stakeholders, including hospital leadership and frontline staff. Studies emphasize the importance of strategic planning and stakeholder engagement to foster a culture receptive to innovation. Without addressing these cultural factors, technological investments risk low adoption and suboptimal utilization [38].

4.4.5 Legal, regulatory, and privacy concerns

The regulatory environment in Iran is still evolving to keep pace with digital health advancements. Legal frameworks governing data privacy, cybersecurity, and ethical use of AI in healthcare are underdeveloped or inconsistently enforced. Concerns about patient data confidentiality and cybersecurity vulnerabilities deter some institutions from fully embracing digital solutions. Research indicates that establishing clear policies and robust data governance structures is critical to building trust and ensuring compliance with international standards. Without such frameworks, hospitals face risks related to data breaches and legal liabilities [39].

4.4.6 Limited maturity of hospital information systems

Evaluations of hospital information systems (HIS) maturity in Iran reveal that most hospitals operate at intermediate stages of digital adoption. According to studies using the Electronic Medical Record Adoption Model (EMRAM), Iranian hospitals typically reach stage 3 out of 7, indicating partial implementation of electronic records and clinical decision support but lacking full integration and optimization. This limited maturity reflects challenges in scaling pilot projects, integrating diverse platforms, and achieving interoperability. The slow pace of HIS development delays the transition to fully smart hospital environments capable of leveraging AI and IoT technologies effectively [40].

4.4.7 Impact of international sanctions

Economic sanctions have indirect but substantial effects on smart hospital implementation by limiting access to advanced medical technologies, software, and international expertise. Sanctions increase costs and complicate procurement processes, which restrict hospitals' ability to upgrade infrastructure and adopt cutting-edge innovations. This external factor uniquely challenges Iran compared to other countries, necessitating tailored strategies to build domestic capabilities and foster local innovation [41].

5. Proposed solutions for smart hospital development

The development of smart hospitals requires a multifaceted approach that integrates advanced technologies, organizational reforms, and strategic policy support. The following key solutions have been identified to successfully build and operate smart hospitals:

5.1 Leveraging advanced digital technologies and big data analytics

One of the primary solutions is the effective use of "Internet + technology" platforms that combine traditional and mobile internet with big data analytics to optimize patient care and hospital operations. A 2024 study demonstrated how integrating barcode, RFID, and 5G networks enables real-time monitoring of critical processes such as digital operating rooms and multidisciplinary consultation centers, reducing medical errors and improving quality of care. Artificial intelligence (AI) technologies, including natural language processing and machine learning, can extract, clean, and analyze large volumes of hospital data to support clinical decision-making, research, and operational efficiency. Establishing hospital-wide Enterprise Resource Planning (ERP) systems and business intelligence (BI) tools facilitates dynamic monitoring of resources, costs, and revenues, enabling smarter management decisions and improved patient satisfaction [42].

5.2 Building robust and inter operable IT infrastructure

Smart hospitals depend on a resilient IT infrastructure capable of supporting high-speed communication, seamless data exchange, and integration of heterogeneous systems. Research highlights the importance of adopting Internet of Things (IoT) architectures that connect sensors, devices, and hospital information systems to enable real-time data collection and analysis. A layered IoT infrastructure model is recommended, addressing data acquisition, transmission, processing, storage, and application layers, each with specific technical requirements and optimization factors. Ensuring interoperability between devices and platforms through adherence to international standards is critical to avoid data silos and enable comprehensive patient monitoring and resource management [34].

5.3 Fostering human-centered design and change management

Successful smart hospital development requires placing human factors at the core of technology implementation. Studies emphasize the need for designing systems that enhance the experiences of patients, clinicians, and administrative staff. This includes intuitive user interfaces, minimizing workflow disruptions, and supporting clinical decision-making without increasing cognitive load. Moreover, change management strategies that involve stakeholder engagement, continuous training, and addressing resistance are essential to facilitate adoption and maximize the benefits of smart technologies. Human-centered approaches also consider ethical implications, data privacy, and maintaining the quality of doctor-patient interactions in increasingly digital environments [34].

5.4 Implementing and sustainable and energy-efficient

Sustainability is increasingly recognized as a vital component of smart hospital development. AI-driven energy management systems can optimize heating, ventilation, air conditioning, and lighting to reduce the environmental impact and operational costs. Experts foresee those smart hospitals will integrate sustainability goals by 2037, balancing technological innovation with energy self-sufficiency and eco-friendly practices. This requires designing hospital buildings equipped with sensors and control systems that monitor environmental conditions and adjust resource use dynamically, contributing to healthier indoor environments and supporting public health objectives [43].

5.5 Developing integrated ecosystems and collaborative business models

Smart hospitals are envisioned as integral parts of broader healthcare ecosystems that include clinics, pharmacies, rehabilitation centers, and home care services. Building interoperable platforms that facilitate data sharing and coordinated care across these entities enhances continuity and quality of care. Research suggests that new service models and business collaborations will emerge by 2027–2032, requiring the joint development of standards and governance frameworks. These ecosystems enable the personalized medicine, remote monitoring, and patient empowerment, transforming the traditional hospital-centric care model into a distributed, patient-centered network [44].

5.6 Promoting policy support, incentives, and interdisciplinary research

Government incentives and supportive policies play a crucial role in accelerating smart hospital adoption. Consolidated interdisciplinary research involving healthcare providers, technology developers, and policymakers is necessary to address challenges related to technology assessment, regulatory compliance, and ethical considerations. Establishing hospital-based health technology assessment (HB-HTA) programs helps evaluate the effectiveness, safety, and cost-efficiency of smart hospital innovations, guiding investment decisions and scaling successful solutions [45].

5.7 Proposed solutions for Smart Hospital Development in Iran

Solutions for Smart Hospital Development in Iran highlight key technological, managerial, and infrastructural aspects. Below is a point-by-point explanation supported by recent scientific literature and case studies:

5.7.1 Adaption of Industry 4.0 technologies

The technologies for smart hospitals include internet of things (IoT), artificial intelligence (AI), blockchain, cloud computing, big data analytics, robotics, augmented and virtual reality, and additive manufacturing. These technologies enable connected and integrated devices that improve patient care, operational efficiency, and reduce time waste. For Iran, investing in local knowledge-based companies and forming joint ventures can overcome sanctions and promote technology adoption [36].

5.7.2 Enhancing hospital information system (HIS)

HIS is fundamental for data integration across administrative and clinical levels, improving healthcare quality and efficiency. Current challenges in Iranian hospitals include lack of clear HIS strategies, poor vendor support, inadequate IT security, and resistance to change.

Solutions involve:

- Developing clear, long-term HIS strategies aligned with the hospital needs
- Selecting vendors with strong local support and standardized systems to ensure interoperability
- Enhancing decision support systems, telemedicine, and staff information systems, which currently score low in Iranian hospitals but are crucial for management and service delivery [46].

5.7.3 Improving services quality and patient-centered care

Smart hospitals focus on improving patient safety, comfort, and early diagnosis through continuous monitoring and data-driven decision-making. Studies show that smart hospital implementation results in better service quality and operational efficiency, which is a priority for Iranian healthcare [47].

5.7.4 Strategic management and policy support

Hospital managers must be trained and equipped to handle smart hospital technologies and processes effectively. Due to Iran's specific challenges such as sanctions and resource limitations, policy support for investment in technology and human resources is critical. Collaboration between the Ministry of Health, medical universities, and private sector can foster the innovation and sustainable development [48].

5.7.5 Addressing legal, privacy, and security concerns

Proper IT security frameworks and privacy protections are essential to safeguard patient data in the smart hospital environments. Developing legal frameworks that support e-health and smart technologies can reduce resistance and build trust among stakeholders [49].

5.7.6 Infrastructure and training

Building the necessary infrastructure for connectivity, data storage, and device integration is a prerequisite. Continuous training and education programs for healthcare staff ensure smooth adoption and utilization of smart technologies [36].

5.7.7 Utilizing data analytics and AI for decision making

Smart hospitals leverage big data and AI to enable predictive analytics, personalized medicine, and efficient resource allocation [50].

6. A successful example of AI application in Hospital Management in Iran: Avaab system (hospital statistics and information system)

The Avaab system, developed by the Ministry of Health and Medical Education of Iran, is a pivotal tool designed to enhance the management and improve efficiency within the healthcare sector, with a specific focus on hospital information management. This web-based, online software platform was commissioned by the Statistics and Information Technology Group of the Hospital Management and Treatment Services Improvement Office in the Ministry of Health. It consolidates, standardizes, and continuously updates hospital statistics and information from all hospitals nationwide, enabling comprehensive and data-driven decision-making [51].

Key features and applications of the Avaab system:

- Data collection on productivity: Avaab collects extensive data on the performance of hospitals, clinics, and healthcare centers. This includes patient volumes, waiting times, resource utilization rates, and service quality indicators.

- Performance analysis and evaluation: The system analyzes the collected data to assess the operational performance of healthcare centers, identifying strengths and weaknesses. These insights facilitate the process improvements and productivity enhancements.

- Reporting and data visualization: Avaab provides diverse, customizable, and visual reports, assisting hospital managers and policymakers in making informed strategic and operational decisions.
- Forecasting and resource planning: By leveraging historical data, Avaab identifies trends and patterns that enable accurate forecasting of future healthcare needs and resource allocation, thereby optimizing human and financial resource management.
- Continuous monitoring and quality improvement: The system offers ongoing performance monitoring of healthcare centers and delivers timely feedback to support continuous quality enhancement of healthcare services.
- Resource management: Through detailed data analysis, Avaab aids in the efficient management of critical resources, including personnel, medical equipment, and pharmaceuticals, helping to minimize the waste and improve utilization.

Overall, the Avaab system plays a crucial role in elevating the quality of healthcare services, increasing operational efficiency, and reducing costs within Iran's health sector. It empowers hospital managers and policymakers with actionable insights derived from real-time data, enabling evidence-based decision-making.

The Avaab system stands as a successful example of artificial intelligence and advanced data analytics applied in hospital management in Iran. By integrating digital technologies and AI-driven analytics, it transforms healthcare management practices, optimizes resource use, and enhances the patient care delivery. This system exemplifies how innovative AI solutions can support healthcare infrastructure development and improve outcomes, positioning Iran as a leader in adopting smart hospital management technologies [51].

7. Conclusion

Hospital management in Iran is at a pivotal crossroads, facing persistent challenges such as financial constraints, workforce shortages, centralized decision-making, and fragmented healthcare delivery. However, the advent of smart hospital technologies—particularly artificial intelligence (AI), internet of things (IoT), and integrated health information systems—offers a transformative pathway toward overcoming these barriers. Evidence from both Iranian and international experiences demonstrates that digital transformation can significantly enhance operational efficiency, resource allocation, and the quality of patient care.

The successful implementation of smart hospitals in Iran requires comprehensive reforms: decentralizing authority, professionalizing hospital leadership, investing in workforce development, and fostering robust integration between public and private sectors. Embracing AI-driven solutions and digital platforms will not only improve clinical outcomes and patient satisfaction but also support sustainable healthcare management in the face of economic and infrastructural limitations. Ultimately, a strategic focus on innovation, capacity building, and evidence-based policy will be essential for Iran to realize the full potential of smart hospitals and ensure resilient, patient-centered healthcare for the future.

Author details

Pir Hossein Kolivand
Health Economics, The University of Shahed, Tehran, Iran

*Address all correspondence to: peirhossein@yahoo.com

References

[1] Tsai TC, Jha AK, Gawande AA, Huckman RS, Bloom N, Sadun R. Hospital board and management practices are strongly related to hospital performance on clinical quality metrics. Health Affairs. 2015;**34**(8):1304-1311

[2] Aboumatar HJ, Chang BH, Al Danaf J, Shaear M, Namuyinga R, Elumalai S, et al. Promising practices for achieving patient-centered hospital care: A national study of high-performing US hospitals. Medical Care. 2015;**53**(9):758-767. DOI: 10.1097/MLR.0000000000000396

[3] Figueroa JF, Feyman Y, Zhou X, Maddox KJ. Hospital-level care coordination strategies associated with better patient experience. BMJ Quality & Safety. 2018;**27**(10):844-851

[4] Albertson EM, Chuang E, O'Masta B, Miake-Lye I, Haley LA, Pourat N. Systematic review of care coordination interventions linking health and social services for high-utilizing patient populations. Population Health Management. 2022;**25**(1):73-85

[5] Buchbinder SB, Thompson JM. Career Opportunities in Health Care Management: Perspectives from the Field. Sudbury, Massachusetts, USA: Jones & Bartlett Publishers; 2010

[6] Pynes JE, Lombardi DN. Human Resources Management for Health Care Organizations: A Strategic Approach. Hoboken, New Jersey, USA: John Wiley & Sons; 2012

[7] Alshareef AG. Hospital management support for patient safety. Disaster and Emergency Medicine Journal. 2025;**10**(1):27-34

[8] Bhagat SV, Kanyal D. Navigating the future: The transformative impact of artificial intelligence on hospital management-a comprehensive review. Cureus. 2024;**16**(2)

[9] Molaei MM, Fatehi M. Digital transformation in health insurance beyond AI and chatbots. Iranian Journal of Health Insurance. 2024;**7**(3):149-160

[10] Amini-Rarani M, Mokhtari S, Akbari M, Zamani Z, Mahdiyan S. Designing Iranian hospital organizational charts: Global comparisons. PLoS One. 2024;**19**(3):e0300985

[11] Emami M, Haghdoost AA, Yazdi-Feyzabadi V, Ahmadi-Gohari M, Mehrolhassani MH. Developing scenarios for the Iranian health system using system dynamics methodology. Health Scope. 2025;**14**(14)

[12] Hosseinabadi N, Badizadeh A, Zaboli R, Nemati A. Challenges and solutions in medical tourism at Iran university of medical sciences: A qualitative study. Medical Journal of The Islamic Republic of Iran (MJIRI). 2025;**39**(1):27-33

[13] Nouri M, Azami S, Ebadi A, Tabrizi JS. Analysis of the structure of public hospitals administration in Iran: A qualitative study. Health Scope. 2021;**10**(2)

[14] Ghiasipour M, Mosadeghrad AM, Arab M, Jaafaripooyan E. Leadership challenges in health care organizations: The case of Iranian hospitals. Medical Journal of the Islamic Republic of Iran. 2017;**31**:96

[15] Saeidifar M, Martini M, Ebrahimzadeh F, Shaygan F, Teli BD, Behzadifar M. Policy brief: Addressing the shortage of human resources in

the Iranian health system. Journal of Preventive Medicine and Hygiene. 2025;**65**(4):E586

[16] Sohrabi R, Tourani S, Jafari M, Joudaki H, Doshmangir L, Moghri J, et al. A scoping review of public hospitals autonomy in Iran: From budgetary hospitals to corporate hospitals. BMC Health Services Research. 2021;**21**:1-6

[17] Chen B, Baur A, Stepniak M, Wang J. Finding the Future of Care Provision: The Role of Smart Hospitals. New York, USA: McKinsey & Company; 2019. p. 31

[18] Halter N. Mayo Clinic Unveils Plans for $5B Campus Expansion. 2023. Available from: https://www.axios.com/local/twin-cities/2023/11/28/mayo-clinic-renderings-5-billion-campus-expansion [Accessed: 6 July 2025]

[19] Xu B, Fang MZ, Zhou Y, Sanaka K, Svensson LG, Grimm RA, et al. Artificial intelligence machine learning based evaluation of elevated left ventricular end-diastolic pressure: A Cleveland Clinic cohort study. Cardiovascular Diagnosis and Therapy. 2024;**14**(5):788

[20] Hopkins EP. Robotics and Telepresence at Johns Hopkins Hospital. Available from: https://ep.jhu.edu/news/robots-making-a-difference-in-healthcare/ [Accessed: 6 July 2025]

[21] Ye J, Hai J, Song J, Wang Z. The role of artificial intelligence in the application of the integrated electronic health records and patient-generated health data. medRxiv. 2024:2024-2005

[22] Aggarwal R, Sounderajah V, Martin G, Ting DS, Karthikesalingam A, King D, et al. Diagnostic accuracy of deep learning in medical imaging: A systematic review and meta-analysis. npj Digital Medicine. 2021;**4**(1):65

[23] Mendhi S, Sawarkar K, Shete A, Vinchurkar K, Mali SS, Singh S, et al. Smart healthcare: Artificial intelligences impact on drug development and patient care. Intelligent Pharmacy. 2025;**1**:45-60

[24] Reis J, Santo PE, Melão N. Impacts of artificial intelligence on public administration: A systematic literature review. In: 2019 14th Iberian Conference on Information Systems and Technologies (CISTI). IEEE; 2019. pp. 1-7.

[25] Vudathaneni VK, Lanke RB, Mudaliyar MC, Movva KV, Kalluri LM, Boyapati R, et al. The impact of telemedicine and remote patient monitoring on healthcare delivery: A comprehensive evaluation. Cureus. 2024;**16**(3)

[26] Ingole P, Baviskar PR, Ghuge M, Dakhare BS, Dongre Y, Dubey P. Optimizing resource allocation in hospitals using predictive analytics and information systems. Journal of Information Systems Engineering and Management. 2025;**10**:400-415

[27] Kumar P. Artificial intelligence (AI)-augmented knowledge management capability and clinical performance: Implications for marketing strategies in health-care sector. Journal of Knowledge Management. 2025;**29**(2):415-441

[28] Dubey A, Tiwari A. Artificial intelligence and remote patient monitoring in US healthcare market: A literature review. Journal of Market Access & Health Policy. 2023;**11**(1):2205618

[29] Angelina Q, Begum K, Kim HC, Tripathy S, Singhal D, Singh S. A structural analysis of AI implementation challenges in healthcare. Algorithms. 2025;**18**(4):189

[30] Rajaei O, Khayami SR, Rezaei MS. Smart hospital definition: Academic and industrial perspective. International Journal of Medical Informatics. 2024;**182**:105304

[31] Levina A, Ilin I, Gugutishvili D, Kochetkova K, Tick A. Towards a smart hospital: Smart infrastructure integration. Journal of Open Innovation: Technology, Market, and Complexity. 2024;**10**(3):100339

[32] Caruso PF, Greco M, Ebm C, Angelotti G, Cecconi M. Implementing artificial intelligence: Assessing the cost and benefits of algorithmic decision-making in critical care. Critical Care Clinics. 2023;**39**(4):783-793

[33] Wasserman L, Wasserman Y. Hospital cybersecurity risks and gaps: Review (for the non-cyber professional). Frontiers in Digital Health. 2022;**4**:862221

[34] Greenhalgh T, Wherton J, Papoutsi C, Lynch J, Hughes G, Hinder S, et al. Beyond adoption: A new framework for theorizing and evaluating nonadoption, abandonment, and challenges to the scale-up, spread, and sustainability of health and care technologies. Journal of Medical Internet Research. 2017;**19**(11):e8775

[35] Shah SD. From innovation to inclusion—Tackling digital equity needs in health care. JAMA Network Open. 2024;**7**(11):e2445334

[36] Golpira R, Tara SM, Raeesi A. Prerequisites of implementing smart hospitals in Iran. Iranian Journal of Culture and Health Promotion. 2023;**7**(2):185-195

[37] Rahimi B, Nadri H, Afshar HL, Timpka T. A systematic review of the technology acceptance model in health informatics. Applied Clinical Informatics. 2018;**9**(03):604-634

[38] Letafatnejad M, Maleki M, Ebrahimi P. Barriers and facilitators of deploying health kiosk in Iran: A qualitative study. Journal of Education and Health Promotion. 2020;**9**(1):95

[39] Soltanian D, Ghahari A. Comparative study of health data security under GDPR and HIPAA: Challenges and implementation opportunities in Iran. Health Law Journal. 2024;**2**(2):1-4

[40] Ayat M, Sharifi M. Maturity assessment of hospital information systems based on electronic medical record adoption model (EMRAM)—Private hospital cases in Iran. International Journal of Communications, Network and System Sciences. 2016;**9**(11):471-477

[41] Kokabisaghi F. Assessment of the effects of economic sanctions on Iranians' right to health by using human rights impact assessment tool: A systematic review. International Journal of Health Policy and Management. 2018;**7**(5):374

[42] Nikzadipanah A, Rahdar M. Industry 4.0 in smart hospital: A scientometric study. Hospital Practices and Research. 2024;**9**(2):437-447

[43] Dolcini M, Brambilla A, Mangili S, Capolongo S. Environmental sustainability in next-generation hospitals. Identifying needs and requirements from healthcare organizations and industry stakeholders. Annali di Igiene: Medicina Preventiva e di Comunita. Sep-Oct 2025;**37**(5):565-573

[44] Jovy-Klein F, Stead S, Salge TO, Sander J, Diehl A, Antons D. Forecasting the future of smart hospitals: Findings from a real-time delphi

study. BMC Health Services Research. 2024;**24**(1):1421

[45] Moro Visconti R, Morea D. Healthcare digitalization and pay-for-performance incentives in smart hospital project financing. International Journal of Environmental Research and Public Health. 2020;**17**(7):2318

[46] Jahanbakhsh M, Sharifi M, Ayat M. The status of hospital information systems in Iranian hospitals. Acta Informatica Medica. 2014;**22**(4):268

[47] Bates DW, Gawande AA. Improving safety with information technology. New England Journal of Medicine. 2003;**348**(25):2526-2534

[48] Doshmangir L, Takian A. Capacity building to improve hospital managers' performance in West Asia. International Journal of Health Policy and Management. 2019;**8**(5):319

[49] Zarei J, Sadoughi F. Information security risk management for computerized health information systems in hospitals: A case study of Iran. Risk Management and Healthcare Policy. 2016;**9**:75-85

[50] Shamsi M. Integrating artificial intelligence for prediction and optimization in hospital management systems (case study: Iranian Hospital in Dubai). Journal of Business and Future Economy. 2024;**1**(4):1-9

[51] Kolivand P, Ayoubzadeh M, Azari S, Rostamniakan S, Ahmadi M, et al. Digital Health. Tehran: Helal Iran Institute of Applied Scientific Higher Education; 2024. 272 p